The 10 Foods
That Should Never
Touch a Woman's Lips

The 10 Foods That Should Never Touch a Woman's Lips

Foods that can damage your health, drain your energy, and interfere with your ability to lose weight

Cristi J. Doll, Ph.D.

(Revised Edition)

Includes: The Busy Woman's Guide to Weight Loss and Fitness

Foreword by: Mark McAfee
Organic Pastures Dairy
Fresno, California

Pink Bow Publishing, Penndel Pennsylvania

Published by: Pink Bow Publishing, USA
www.pinkbowpublishing.com
ISBN 0-9771588-0-2

Cover Design by: Irene Archer
Archer Graphics
Irene@book-cover-design.com

Library of Congress Card Number 2005907689

Disclaimer

The purpose of this book is to educate and expand the reader's knowledge about nutrition and fitness, and is not rendering medical advice, nor has it been evaluated by the FDA. Before beginning any new diet or exercise program it is strongly advised that you consult a physician. The information contained in this book is not intended to replace any advice or treatment that may have been prescribed by your physician. The publisher, author, or advisors are in no way responsible for any physical, mental, emotional, or financial harm caused or alleged to be caused directly or indirectly by following any part, section, advice, or suggestion, found in this book. All forms of exercise pose some inherent risk, and thus the reader is advised to take full responsibility for his or her personal safety and not perform exercises beyond his or her level of fitness, experience, or ability. If you do not agree with the above, you may return this book to the publisher for a full refund.

This book is dedicated to:

Mom and Dad
I love you more then anything in this world.

My son, Steven
If I could reach the stars, I'd give them all to you.

Mom and Pop
Your spirits are with me every day.

My husband, Christopher
It's about the love!

Acknowledgements

I would like to begin with acknowledging the two people who put so much time, love, and energy into this project.

First, my husband *Christopher* who spent countless hours reading and rereading this book as it developed from draft to draft. Thank you for your unwavering dedication to this project whose message is clearly reflected in the life we lead as a couple: simple, pure, and real. Thank you for helping me live the life of my dreams..."It's about the love!"

Secondly, I would like to say thank you to *Mark McAfee* for the heartfelt words that open this book. Your passion and dedication to helping people reclaim their health through knowledge and access to live foods is a message America's women need to hear. Your words bring tears to my eyes, humility to my heart, and encourage me to keep spreading the message that the weight loss and health fix millions of women are searching for is not found in a pill or the latest diet, it is found at the nearest organic farm, organic food store, or farmer's market.

Finally, I would like to thank the family members, teachers, and mentors who helped instill in me the passion for physical fitness and healthy living that I now share with others.

Table of Contents

Foreword.. xi

About This Book... xvii

Introduction.. xix

Chapter 1...1
The 10 Foods That Should Never
Touch a Woman's Lips

Chapter 2...39
Lost in a Toxic Cloud of Dietary Confusion

Chapter 3...51
I Would Love to Eat Right But...

Chapter 4...57
Coming Out of the Clouds:
Learning to Recognize Real Foods

Chapter 5...69
Healthy Meals for Busy Women

Chapter 6...103
The Busy Woman's Guide to Weight Loss and Fitness

Letters from Readers...113

Parting Thoughts..116

Thoughts of a Raw Organic Dairy Farmer
By: Mark McAfee

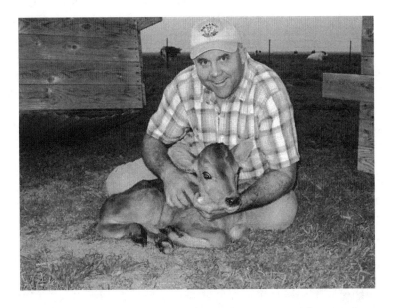

As fate would have it, my 16 years spent in paramedic medicine evolved into a lifetime commitment to health. I pursued my passion with an even greater purpose after I retired and took over management of my family's farms.

In founding the first and only organic, pasture-fed raw dairy and creamery in the US, I now find myself in the midst of (and occasionally leading) a grass roots, people initiated raw revolution; a diverse, nation-wide community demanding access to living, whole foods. The impact of this movement touches every part of our world. Citizens across this great nation are awaking to the fact that the food supply they are being offered by factory farms and corporate America is not enzyme rich, not bio-diverse or whole....it is making them fat and sick. These great American brands (including most organic products) are enzyme depleted, biologically dead, preserved, and are Ultra High Temperature processed to provide long shelf life, homogenized, standardized, pasteurized, oxidized and sterilized.

Given the nature (or lack thereof) of our food supply, it is no wonder that Americans are over-weight and immune depressed. Immune systems are supported and strengthened when biologically living foods are consumed. The goal of ESL (extended shelf life technology) is primarily to kill any living thing that might wish to live in the food packaging. If something starts to live in our food products then it might change the flavor, color, consistency, or "mouth feel" modern food science has invested so heavily in creating. Spoilage is anti-profit. For a food product to compete on crowded and competitive market shelves, its producers must design it to enter into a national distribution system and have a long shelf-life. All products must be very dead and very preserved.

An ever-increasing monoculture pervades modern American society extending to our concept of medicine, the way we fuel our cars, housing, schooling, modern farming practices, processing technologies, and even our politics. If it conflicts with our beliefs, does not speak our language, shoots back when challenged, if it is alive in a package, if it has bacteria (good or bad), if it is an insect that makes a small scar on our fruit, if it does not make an unnaturally massive amount of milk….then give it antibiotics, spray it with pesticides, inject it with hormones, genetically modify it, radiate it, sterilize it, sanction it, ban it, jail it on an island, deny it rights, suppress it, bomb it, kill it; we make no space for it. Food values are just one symptom of our nations gathering illness; an illness that pervades all levels of our society.

It was not always this way. Our land was settled into small agrarian, self-sufficient communities. Citizens were close to the soil and knew and trusted the farmer. Food was fresh, enzyme rich, lacto-fermented, bio-diverse, whole and unprocessed. This was the food of our ancestors. As we have moved away from the farm, we no longer have a connection to the land and we do not understand the value of food or whole nutrition.

Now, Americans seeking this lost connection must find an organic farmer or go to Whole Foods and spend their "entire pay check" to get food that is whole, unprocessed, raw, antibiotic free, pesticide free, organic, fair trade and socially conscious. These foods can be expensive, rare and politically incorrect. These foods prevent disease, extend our lives, taste great...and build our immune systems. Most states ban access to raw foods, especially raw milk. Health-conscience consumers seeking raw milk outside of California either find a local black market source or buy from OPDC on the internet at $32 dollars per gallon, delivered overnight by UPS with cold packs. This defines crazy; but not when the milk assists the body in effectively relieving or eliminating such conditions as Osteoporosis, Asthma and Arthritis. Things will change; it is just a matter of time.

It would probably appear from a celestial observer's point of view that we Americans are a bunch of sheep that have no idea what the truth is...that we are lost and going in big circles...saying one thing and doing another... our opinions are led by the media, corporate advertisements and the NASDAQ stock value. The most odious may be the "Happy California Cow" commercials depicting cows flirting with each other even showing a bovine sex drive while on grass pastures. There are virtually no cows on pastures in California and they are nearly 100% artificially inseminated. They live on big piles of manure or on flushed concrete floors being milked three times per day. When consumers challenged these ads as false advertising, the case was thrown out because the advertiser, the California Milk Advisory Board was granted immunity from these kinds of legal challenges. Beware, we are being brain washed and soon we will have no reference to the truth.

In the same light, one of my favorite political diseases is lactose intolerance. The disease condition and diagnosis created by man to excuse the deficiencies made by pasteurizing milk. Humans have no lactose intolerance to raw milk (raw milk contains all of the required bacterial cultures and enzymes required for digestion). Pretty soon diseases will be blamed on human deficiencies and not the processed foods that are their true origin. What a convenient way to sell more drugs to healthy people.

It is essential that each and every one of us find the inner truth and find our own true north. The studies conducted by Weston A. Price pointed the direction 70 years ago, when he discovered the facts behind "not so obvious modern disease patterns". He found that primitive cultures did not suffer from modern diseases. However, as soon as these primitive cultures started eating modern processed foods they began to suffer a broad range of modern diseases including cancers and immune depression.

We now suffer from ADD, autism, heart disease, cancers, diabetes, erectile dysfunction, antibiotic-resistant "superbug" bacterial infections... these things where unheard of 125 years ago. It seems that the longer the list of diagnoses we suffer from, the more drugs can be made to address these diseases. We Americans do not have a health care system; we have a sick care system. When was the last time you heard of a healthy person going to the doctor to get a medication or a surgery? Sick people make money, healthy people do not. Mankind seems to be its own worst enemy.

I mix and blend the discussion of politics, nutrition, and power all together in these words not because I am confused but because I am not confused. This is space ship earth with one huge ecosystem and 6 billion souls with matching inner ecosystems. There is a raw revolution going on, a revolution of truth and consumer empowerment. We must question the FDA and "paid-for science." Drugs have a limited place in our lives. A much greater place belongs to our primary diet and the right to access unprocessed whole foods.

As a farmer, I am forever blessed by contact with my customers. This sacred relationship is mostly missing in today's American culture. A great circle is about to be complete. As Americans discover that the foods being sold to them at the store are the origin of their disease or immune depression, they will be forced to find a farmer, just as our ancestors did.

There are certain things that should not pass by a woman's lips. However, what should come out from a woman's lips is a much longer list. Kisses, a voice for freedom and loving words are just the beginning. Women are the passionate voice for change. The majority of visitors at Organic Pastures Dairy are breast feeding women and their children getting an education about nutrition. Women nourish the world and bring life, love, and peace.

I am one man that encourages women to take a choke hold on the direction of this country and this world one bite, one swallow, and one hug at a time. Do not ever underestimate the power of a passionate, educated mother and her desire to feed her family according to her beliefs. Nothing will stop her when she knows that the health of her family is hanging in the balance.

When a family is healthy, warm, well fed and loved...all is well.

Join the raw revolution...only living food brings life!

Mark McAfee
Founder
Organic Pastures Dairy Company

About This Book

This book is about the foods millions of women eat every day that can damage their health, drain their energy, and interfere with their ability to lose weight. My purpose in writing this book is to help women make the connection between their daily food choices and their current health. Years of neglecting to supply the body with essential nutrients can contribute to a host of nagging and debilitating health problems including: chronic fatigue, sinus infections, cancer, diabetes, gastrointestinal problems, arthritis, weight gain, and reproductive issues.

Within these pages is an overview of what I believe are the *key players;* that is, the collection of foods I see as the strongest contributors to these conditions. Individually, these foods are bad for a woman's health; collectively, they are a disaster. My challenge is to convince you against the tide of ever-present and deceptive marketing campaigns by those peddling processed foods, that these 10 foods should in fact be limited or avoided altogether

Such deceptive marketing creates what I refer to as, "A Toxic Cloud of Dietary Confusion." This cloud fogs women's perception, interferes with their ability to recognize and choose healthy foods, and keeps them ensnared in destructive eating patterns. The longer they stay lost in this toxic cloud of confusion, the farther they move away from achieving the healthy, energetic, lean bodies they desire.

Fortunately, once this toxic cloud has been lifted, it becomes much easier for women to recognize that the weight loss and health fix they are searching for is not found in a pill or the latest diet; it is found at the nearest farm, natural food store, and farmer's market.

May this book reacquaint you with food's true place in your life.

Introduction

Man has been living off what the land provides him since time began. Plants and animals indigenous to his area served him well until the past few generations when he began to interfere with his food supply and the natural order within him became disrupted.

The hunter-fisher-gatherer diet consisted of wild plant foods (such as fruits, nuts, seeds, leaves and stems), insects, some milk, and the meat, organs, and marrow of wild animals and fish. It has been only within the past 10,000 years, since the advent of agriculture, that grains, legumes, and dairy byproducts have had a standard place in the human diet.

The change from aboriginal diets to the modern Western diet can be followed as man began to form villages. His life became less mobile as he began to cultivate and store foods that could feed large numbers of people. Early agricultural communities began to raise crops that would grow well in their area and supplemented their diet with animals that could be killed close to the settlement.

Over time, those with the responsibility for providing food for the growing community learned to domesticate animals and plants which had once only been hunted and gathered. Wild grains quickly gained a place in the diets of both man and his newly domesticated animals. A sufficient amount of stored food was necessary for the survival of the newly forming urban civilizations. A plentiful food supply meant the settlement survived; conversely, when food was scarce health declined and disease followed. Frequently it became necessary for a settlement to relocate.

As agricultural practices developed, it was no longer necessary for man to spend most of his time in the pursuit of food. Agriculture brought man a semblance of stability and a sense of security he had never known before. In fact, his diet and way of life gradually improved over the next 10,000 years as a result of agriculture and domesticated animals.

The agricultural diet maintained many elements of the traditional hunter-gatherer-fisher diet. Fresh meat from free-ranging domestic animals and fish for coastal and river people were a staple in addition to nuts, fresh vegetables and fruits. Raw milk and dairy products, along with whole grains added other sources of nutrients and were consumed by agricultural societies everywhere for thousands of years. Whether one ate more in the manner of the hunter-fisher-gatherer, or that of the agriculturist, there was a wide spectrum of foods to build healthy bodies.

Although animals in the wild and those within hunter-fisher-gatherer communities are not immune to disease, the incidence rate of chronic and degenerative disease in both populations is very low. However, once animals and people begin to assimilate non-traditional and commercially manufactured foods the incidence of such diseases increases sharply.

When modern foods: white breads, jams, canned vegetables, vegetable oils, syrup, chocolate and coffee became widely available, the health of those consuming these foods quickly began to change. As advances in transportation made the world much smaller and easier to navigate, food storage, preservation, and distribution quickly improved. This made it much easier and economical for processed food manufactures to get their products into the hands of consumers around the world. We had moved from a world where most everyone grew, prepared, and consumed a diet based on "whole" foods into a world where the foods we now eat are grown possibly far away and have likely been processed before being transported to local merchants.

Today in the United States, what we eat has changed more in the last forty years then in the previous forty-thousand. Americans are clearly the most overfed yet undernourished nation in the world as even the most cursory statistic will show. The Standard American Diet has strayed far from the whole-food diet of our ancestors of just a few generations ago. Sadly, as Americans get fatter and continue consuming meals of nutrient-deficient processed food, they begin to get sick.

One can only guess how much is spent each year in this country treating diet related illnesses. Birth defects, learning disabilities, hyperactivity, arthritis, ulcers, mental illness, osteoporosis, allergies, and chronic fatigue are only a small list in the litany of degenerative diseases and disorders linked to improper diet that are sapping the life-blood of our nation.

Unfortunately, even with such overwhelming evidence linking diet to health, this is not news most people want to hear; nor is it information the commercial food industry wants you to be concerned with. After all, commercial foods are big business and business is concerned with making money, not protecting health. Today, most popular diets and those offering nutritional guidelines turn a blind eye to the devitalizing effects processed foods are having on the health of our nation.

Chapter 1

The 10 Foods
That Should Never Touch
a Woman's Lips

The ten foods that should never touch a woman's lips are not individual foods per se, but food categories such as processed foods or food ingredients like artificial sweeteners. Individually, these foods can be damaging to a women's health; collectively, they can be a disaster.

1. Table Salt

2. Refined Flour

3. Refined Sugars

4. Artificial Sweeteners

5. Damaged Fats

6. Modern Milk and Dairy Products

7. Caffeine

8. Processed Meats

9. Processed Food

10. Fast Food

The 1st Food
That Should Never Touch a Woman's Lips

Table Salt

Salt is absolutely essential to human health. Salt alkalizes blood and other vital fluids, stabilizes water balance, plays an important role in the functions of the nervous system, aids in digestion and elimination, and is deeply involved in the biochemistry of metabolism. Excess salt however, can contribute to such conditions as stomach cancer, acid reflux, PMS, headaches, calcium loss, hyperactivity, insomnia, and hypertension.

The 1,500 mg to 2,000 mg of sodium necessary to meet daily human nutritional needs can and should be obtained from fruits, vegetables, and the occasional use sea salt. Regrettably, most of the sodium Americans get comes from *processed foods* which contain high quantities of refined salt. A single serving of most canned soups for example, contains around 900 mg of salt per serving.

What do I mean by refined salt? During processing, regular table salt is stripped of virtually all naturally occurring minerals and trace elements including magnesium. Magnesium is essential for proper immune function, proper performance of nerve and brain cells, and is involved in the metabolism of sugars and fats. Additionally, dextrose (sugar) is often added to regular table salt to eliminate the bitter taste resulting from being chemically cleaned and bleached.

Processed table salt has other ingredients that have no place in a healthy diet, specifically anti-caking agents which prevent the salt from mixing with water in the shaker. Thus, table salt does not dissolve effectively inside our bodies; instead, it builds up in the organs and tissues which can lead to severe health problems. Consumed daily, table salt, refined and denatured for convenience and higher profits, undermines rather than supports health.

What's a Girl to Do?

The majority of your diet should consist of fresh foods. This will help insure that the nutrients you receive are naturally occurring, and not added during processing. If you do select packaged foods read the labels carefully, and consider shopping for these products at a local natural food store in your area. These stores generally have a nice selection of higher quality packaged foods that tend to be free of dangerous additives and preservatives, and often use sea salt instead of table salt.

In our house we use Redmond's Real Salt. Redmond's contains over 50 naturally occurring trace minerals including iodine. Unlike table salt, it is not heated, bleached, or altered with chemicals. You can read more about sea salt at www.realsalt.com.

The 2nd and 3rd Foods
That Should Never Touch a Woman's Lips

Refined Flour and Sugar: The Evil Twins

Refined flour and refined sugars are integral parts of the Standard American Diet. Rarely is one consumed without the other. I place refined flour on an equal level with refined sugar with regard to its damaging effects on health, as void of all or most of its fiber and inherent nutritional properties after processing, refined flour is easily converted into sugar by the body. Thus, I have decided to present them together as they are co-conspirators in so many of the health problems facing women today:

mood swings	hyperactivity
indigestion	heart disease
kidney stones	fatigue
vaginal yeast infections	emotional problems
osteoporosis	hormone imbalance
liver dysfunction	colitis
menstrual problems	Arthritis
cancer	food cravings
allergies	high estrogen levels
drug, caffeine, and food	PMS
addictions	impaired immunity
anxiety	high blood pressure
diabetes	high triglyceride levels
asthma	bloating
tooth decay	adrenal exhaustion
ulcers	depression
sinus infections	congestion

Most women underestimate how bad refined flour and sugar actually are for them. Sugar related health problems are far reaching and well documented:

- High insulin levels are linked to: cardiovascular disease (high triglyceride levels, low HDL levels)

- Cancer (cancer cells feed directly on sugar)

- Adult onset diabetes (almost entirely diet related)

- Hypoglycemia (the pancreas reacting to excess processed carbohydrates by sending so much insulin that blood sugar drops)

- Excess sugar can interfere with the body's ability to withstand disease.

Sadly, few women make the connection between their daily food choices and their health and weight challenges. This is particularly true with regard to refined flours and sugars, the foods women often choose to increase their energy throughout the day (bagels, donuts, crackers, pastries, pop tarts, candy, soda, energy bars, processed fruit drinks). Such forms of fuel (carbohydrates) are indeed the body's primary source of food energy in addition to proteins and fats. However, the refining process strips once whole grains, fruits, and vegetables of their vital nutrients transforming them into "empty or negative" calorie sources that actually deplete the body of vital nutrient reserves. Our bodies simply were not designed to consume the large sum of processed carbohydrates that millions of Americans eat every day.

Carbohydrates from fruits, starchy vegetables, and whole grains as found in Nature, whole and unrefined, are nutritionally beneficial. They provide natural energy to help

5

energize our bodies and brains. These real foods have been nourishing people for thousands of years.

One must note that refined sugars were not used in great quantities until the 20th century. The latest statistics from the U.S. Census Bureau, Statistical Abstract of the United States: 2004-2005, shows that Americans consume on average nearly 150 lbs of sugars per year. Unfortunately, in an attempt to cut down on their consumption of sugars, many women turn to artificial sweeteners. As you will read in the following section, artificial sweeteners are no panacea.

Avoid Foods Containing
the Following Forms of Sugar

raw sugar	corn syrup solids
brown sugar	cane juice crystals
powdered sugar	sorghum syrup
white-sugar (sucrose)	glucose solids
maltodextrin	lactose
caramel	mannitol
beet sugar	refiner's syrup
barley malt	sorbitol
fructose	xylitol
maltose	dextrose
carob syrup	

*****high fructose corn syrup*****

What's a Girl to Do?

Read labels carefully when selecting grain products. Most processed bagels, cereals, pasta, breads, rolls, pastries, and cookies have been overly refined and derived from grains grown with pesticides, fertilizers, and fungicides. Additionally, these low quality foods also contain a variety of sweeteners and synthetic vitamins, along with an array of artificial flavors, colors, and preservatives.

Ingredients:
Wonder White Bread

Enriched wheat flour [flour, barley malt, ferrous sulfate (iron), "B" vitamins (niacin, thiamine mononitrate (B1), riboflavin (B2), folic acid)], water, high fructose corn syrup, yeast, contains 2% or less of: soybean oil, salt, calcium sulfate, wheat gluten, soy flour, dough conditioners (may contain: sodium stearoyl lactylate, calcium dioxide, calcium iodate, diammonium phosphate, di-calcium phosphate, monocalcium phosphate, mono and diglycerides, ethoxylated mono and diglycerides, calcium

Ingredients:
Orowheat 100% Whole Wheat Bread

Whole wheat flour, water, high fructose corn syrup, cracked wheat, honey, wheat gluten, salt, yeast, soybean oil, molasses, wheat bran, raisin juice concentrate, calcium proprionate (preservative), grain vinegar, sodium stearoyl lactylate, monoglycerides, calcium sulfates, ascorbic acid (dough conditioner), soy lecithin, azodicarbonamide.

Fortunately, with the overwhelming growth of stores like Whole Foods Markets, savvy health conscious consumers are demanding higher quality foods. As a result, many neighborhood grocery stores are beginning to carry a variety of organic and natural foods. By simply reading the labels, you will quickly see a noticeable difference between organic sprouted-grain breads for example, and the highly processed breads I listed above. My favorite bread is Nature's Path Organic Manna Bread; go to www.naturespath.com for more information. My husband and I eat so much of this delicious bread that I order it by the case and keep extra loaves in the freezer. It is available in several delicious varieties.

Here are the ingredients for Nature's Path Multi-Grain Manna Bread:

Sprouted Organic Whole Wheat Kernels, Filtered Water, Organic Brown Rice, Organic Barley, Organic Millet, Organic Flax Seed, Organic Rye Kernels, Organic Soya Beans, Organic Rolled Oats, Organic Oat Bran, and Organic Corn Meal.

We also buy French Meadow brand organic breads. Here are the ingredients for their "summer" loaf:

Stone-ground organic wheat flour with the wheat germ, stone-ground organic wheat flour, pure water, unrefined sea salt.

Avoid breads that contain synthetic vitamins (a sure sign the flour has been overly refined), high fructose corn syrup and other refined sugars; along with artificial flavors, colors, and preservatives.

The 4th Food
That Should Never Touch a Woman's Lips

Artificial Sweeteners

Artificial sweeteners can be found in stores across America including health food stores, within products frequently labeled as, "sugar-free, low-sugar, light, diet, diabetic, or reduced-calorie." In the United States, artificial sweeteners are known under such trade names as: Equal® and NutraSweet® for (aspartame), Splenda® for (sucralose), and Sweet-n-Low® (saccharine).

Artificial sweeteners win the prize for being the most health damaging food product passed off as healthy (or at least generally regarded as safe) by both government agencies and food manufacturers. Deceptive marketing campaigns and studies conducted by groups determined to profit from these substances, have effectively convinced millions of women attempting to reduce their sugar intake that artificial sweeteners are the feel-good, *healthy* alternative for them and their families. Nothing could be farther from the truth.

Aspartame

Aspartame was approved by the FDA for use in foods in 1981 and in carbonated beverages in 1983. Adverse reactions from aspartame reported to the US Food and Drug Administration include: headaches, dizziness, seizures, nausea, numbness, muscle spasms, weight gain, rashes, depression, fatigue, irritability, tachycardia, insomnia, vision problems, hearing loss, heart palpitations, breathing difficulties, anxiety attacks, slurred speech, loss of taste, tinnitus, vertigo, memory loss, and joint pain.

Conditions such as hypoglycemia, brain tumors, epilepsy, chronic fatigue syndrome, Alzheimer's, multiple sclerosis, birth defects and diabetes can be triggered or made worse by aspartame according to researcher and neurosurgeon Russell Blaylock, author of Excitotoxins: The Taste That Kills (Health Press, 1997), as use of aspartame kills nerve cells which can trigger or worsen such conditions.

Furthermore, aspartame can increase cravings for carbohydrates and sugars, the exact things women turn to artificial sweeteners to avoid. What sparks these cravings is one of aspartame's components, phenylalaline, which can block the production of serotonin in the brain. When production of serotonin is disrupted, a variety of symptoms can be triggered including depression and PMS in addition to an increase in sugar and carbohydrate cravings

Saccharin

Saccharin is in the sugar substitute Sweet-n- Low®, which is found in those little pink packets on the tables of restaurants across America. Saccharin is the controversial ingredient found to cause bladder cancer in male lab rats and an increased risk of bladder cancer in humans. As a result, in 1977 the Food and Drug Administration (FDA) required that any food containing saccharin have labels that warn consumers about potential hazards to their health. The labels said: *"Use of this product may be hazardous to your health. This product contains saccharin, which has been determined to cause cancer in laboratory animals."* Researchers however, argued that those consuming saccharine in moderation did not have a greater risk of developing bladder cancer then anyone else. Thus, in 2000, the government removed saccharine from the list of known carcinogens.

I believe that as long as manufactures are making money from saccharine or any of the other artificial sweeteners currently available, there will always be scientific evidence to support both sides depending on who's doing the experiment. Is it really worth the risk?

Sucralose:
What I have affectionately nicknamed...
swimming pool sugar

The sweetness of Splenda® is derived from a chlorocarbon chemical that contains three atoms of chlorine in every one of its molecules. The manufacturer of this chlorinated compound named it sucralose. These chlorine molecules make sucralose 600 times sweeter than a natural molecule of sugar which contains no chlorine.

To date, there have been no long-term human studies on Splenda® to determine the potential health effects on people. Hence, no one can say with certainty that the substance is safe to eat. And, as with aspartame, sucralose can cause a variety of side effects.

According to Dr. Marcelle Pick, OB/GYN in an article she wrote for her Woman to Woman website titled, "Splenda®-is it safe, or truly the perfect artificial sweetener?" some of the side effects that have been observed in humans consuming products containing sucralose include skin rashes, dizziness, intestinal cramping, headaches, stomach pain, bladder issues, panic-like agitation, diarrhea, and muscle aches.

Dr. Pick goes on to explain how artificial sweeteners are a classic example of bait and switch. According to Dr. Pick, artificial sweeteners entice the brains receptor cells into thinking it is about to receive something sweet. When the sweet food never arrives, you might feel a sudden craving for carbohydrates since the brain is still awaiting the energy boost that follows sweet foods. Finally, Dr. Pick explains that this is why so many diet beverage manufacturers add caffeine to such products so that the brain gets rewarded with the "jolt" you promised it.

The effects that artificial sweeteners might have are determined by each person's individual biochemistry. As with cigarettes, it might take years of daily doses of artificial sweeteners for a resulting disease to occur. By then however, you are already sick.

What's a Girl to Do?

Many women think that since a product does not contain sucrose (table sugar) it must be better for their health, and will assist them in losing weight. Sadly, few women ever consider that they are simply replacing one product that poses both immediate and long-term health risks, with another product that poses both immediate and long-term health risks. Although I strongly discourage the use of refined sugars, I would eat a cookie containing regular sugar long before I would eat one laced with any artificial sweetener.

If you or someone you love frequently consumes products containing artificial sweeteners, I strongly suggest that you obtain copies of the following books and review the web sites listed below, as artificial sweeteners can result in a wide range of side effects from mild to severe. A study of available literature suggests that the public is at great risk from repeated exposure to artificial sweeteners. Serious consideration should be given to discontinuing the use of products containing aspartame (Equal® and NutraSweet®), sucralose (Splenda®), and saccharine (Sweet and Low®).

- Russell Baylock's, Excitotoxins: The Taste That Kills (Health Press, Santa Fe, Mew Mexico, c1994).

- Mary Nash Stoddard's <u>Deadly Deception - Story of Aspartame</u> (Odenwald Press 1998).
- <u>www.aspartamesafety.com</u>

- <u>www.aspartame.com</u>

Question: Are there any sweeteners that are OK for women to consume and offer to their families?

Answer: With the obvious overuse of sugars in America I am always hesitant to recommend any sweeteners because far too many will ignore my pleas for consumption in moderation. Life should be sweet, but far too many of us are drowning in excess sugar.

Here are the sweeteners I use:

- organic fruit (fresh, frozen, or dried)
- yams, sweet potatoes, and pumpkin
- spices such as cinnamon, nutmeg, and cloves
- pure vanilla extract
- raw honey
- 100% maple syrup
- Rapunzel Rapadura™ (unrefined and unbleached dried organic whole cane sugar) <u>www.rapunzel.com</u>
- Sucanat (evaporated organic sugar cane juice)
- molasses
- coconut

The 5ᵗʰ Food
That Should Never Touch a Woman's Lips

Damaged Fats

No matter how often women might hear that a certain amount of fat in their diet is necessary for their bodies to work properly, they continued to avoid such foods as nuts, olives, coconut, red meat, avocado, and whole fat dairy products including butter. Rarely do they consider that avoidance of such nutrient dense whole foods might be the reason they cannot get pregnant, are always hungry, their skin is dry, their hormones are not balanced, and their hair is falling out. These foods have been nourishing people for thousands of years before processed food manufacturers began replacing them with low cost, highly processed fats and fat alternatives.

Processed food manufactures have convinced women (those who purchase most of the family's food), that these "new" fats are not only less expensive, but better for their health.

At the turn of the 20ᵗʰ century, most of the fat in the American diet was saturated or monounsaturated and came from butter, lard, coconut oils, olive oil, as well as meat and whole milk. One should note that obesity and the vast array of degenerative diseases spreading across this country today were extremely rare even 50 years ago although people consumed what they are told today are "bad fats" that should be avoided. Today, most of the fats Americans consume are polyunsaturated, primarily from vegetable oils.

The problem with polyunsaturated oils is that they tend to oxidize and go rancid when subjected to heat, oxygen, and moisture when they are cooked and processed. In her book, Nourishing Traditions (New Trends Publishing, 2001), author Sally Fallon states that these damaged fats

14

behave as "marauders" in the body for they attack cell membranes and red blood cells. She goes on to say that such free-radical damage can cause the skin to wrinkle prematurely, and can set the stage for tumors as these free-radicals damage the tissues and organs. Free-radical damage to the blood vessels initiates the buildup of plaque in the arteries.

Furthermore, commercial processing of these oils causes a disruption in the balance of omega-3 and omega-6 linolenic acids. This disruption creates an imbalance in the body which has been linked to blood clots, high blood pressure, digestive irritation, sterility, depressed immune function, cancer, and weight gain.

Processed oils are obtained by either extraction or hydrogenation. In the past, extraction was achieved by slow moving stone presses. Today, extraction of oils occurs in large factories that crush the oil-bearing seeds exposing them to extremely high temperatures in addition to damaging light and oxygen. This process breaks down the fatty-acids creating free-radicals and destroys valuable nutrients, especially vitamin E.

The other process that turns polyunsaturated oils into a more usable form for processed foods is called hydrogenation. In the early 1900's American chemists began using cheap vegetable oils to produce a substitute for butter and came up with margarine and shortening. They did this by heating the vegetable oil to over 500° F, then pumping hydrogen through it and adding nickel as a catalyst to harden it. The result is a solid fat substitute with a molecular structure very similar to plastic. Strong emulsifiers are added to give it a thick consistency, and unpleasant odors are removed with bleach. Dyes and flavorings must then be added so that the product resembles something palatable.

These damaged fats are promoted as health foods, a marketing triumph as can be seen in the popularity of margarine, shortening, vegetable oils, and other butter substitutes. Partially hydrogenated oils are even more dangerous then other commercially processed oils because of the chemical changes that occur during hydrogenation. Furthermore, these *trans fats* are known to significantly lower good cholesterol (HDL) and significantly increase bad cholesterol (LDL). Consumption of these hydrogenated fats has been associated with a variety of chronic illnesses and conditions including cancer, birth defects, diabetes, heart disease, sterility, difficulty in lactation, problems with bones and tendons, along with obesity and depressed immune function.

In an article titled, "Trans Fats 101," from the University of Maryland's web site, Registered Dietician Cynthia Payne writes, "Trans fats increase the risk for heart disease. Therefore, children who start at age 3 or 4 eating a steady diet of fast food, pop tarts, commercially prepared fish sticks, stick margarine, cake, candy, cookies, and microwave popcorn can be expected to get heart disease earlier then kids who are eating foods without trans fats."

Ladies, I encourage you to avoid using vegetable oils including soy, corn, cotton seed, and canola, along with hydrogenated and partially hydrogenated oils. If you avoid processed foods, this will be very easy.

What's a Girl to Do?

The inclusion of healthy fats in your diet is essential for good health. Do not equate fresh nuts, avocados, and olives with the obesity epidemic sweeping this country. Americans are not getting fat from eating too many walnuts or avocados; America is however getting fat from eating too much junk food. I encourage you to include plenty of traditional fats and oils including butter, avocado, raw nuts and nut butters, macadamia nut oil, olive oil, flax oil, and coconut oil. Look for "cold-pressed" or "expeller pressed" on the label. Use healthy fats in your diet each day; your hair, skin, nails, and hormones will thank you for it.

The 6th Food
That Should Never Touch a Woman's Lips

Modern Milk

Since dairy foods were not frequently part of the traditional hunter-gatherer diet, not everyone agrees that milk should be consumed by humans after infancy. This argument states that since no other species drinks milk after weaning, neither should we. Yes, millions of years of evolution have shown that once weaned, humans can live healthy lives without milk. However, over the past 10,000 years raw milk products have played a major role in building healthy bodies.

With the advent of agriculture, raw milk products became a staple in many parts of the world. Many healthy nomadic and agricultural societies have depended on milk from cattle, sheep, goats, horses, water buffalo, and camels for their animal protein and fat. As groups of people roamed less, they hunted less. Milk replaced animal bones as the chief source of calcium and other minerals. The primary difference between the pasteurized milk products of today and those consumed by our ancestors is that the milk once came from pasture fed animals that grazed throughout the year on live grass, while most dairy cows today are raised in pens and fed processed grains. The quality of the milk depends on the health of the animals it comes from and was never in question until the animals began being raised in stalls and fed grains and other food sources instead of the grass from green pastures. As the quality of the milk changed so did the health of those consuming its byproducts.

In the United States, the heating of milk to high temperatures to kill pathogens in milk began about 120-150 years ago as millions of people (mostly within the inner-cities) died from diseases transmitted from raw milk.

Young children were particularly susceptible. Low-quality milk produced by dairies in the inner cities of New York and Boston for example, denied their cows access to pasture for grazing. Instead, they stood around in manure in cramped quarters and were fed "brewer's mash," a very low-quality feed, which resulted in very low-quality milk that was low in protein, mineral, and fat content, and full of dangerous pathogens.

During this same period in history, milk producers did not have access to refrigeration, or to milking equipment that could be effectively sanitized. What resulted was rampant disease that killed millions. The spreading of disease through low-quality milk ended when dairies began to heat milk to high temperatures.

The success of pasteurization launched the commercial dairy industry as producers began to pool their milk. Although the quality of the milk that resulted was very poor, profits increased and no one died. Such practices continue today with the main advantage being "extend-shelf-life."

What is interesting to note here is that milk from the countryside taken from clean, healthy, pasture grazed cows was considered the best medicine of the day. In fact, respected medical clinics in the past depended on high quality raw milk to help treat many diseases.

In addition to destroying helpful organisms, pasteurization does much more to denature milk. It destroys heat-liable nutrients such as vitamin C and vitamin B_{12}, changing the chemical structures of proteins and fats in the milk. Furthermore, pasteurization destroys all the enzymes in milk; in fact, the test for successful pasteurization is the absence of enzymes. These enzymes help the body assimilate all body building factors, including calcium. That is why those who drink pasteurized milk may suffer from osteoporosis. Once all of the nutritional value has been stripped from the milk by pasteurization, synthetic vitamin D_2, D_3 and colors are added. Since most dairy cows are no longer grazed outdoors in the sun they are unable to absorb natural vitamin D. As a result, the bright yellow color in butter disappears, a clear sign that vitamin D and carotenes are no longer present. Hence, dairy manufacturers add yellow dye to restore color in butter and powdered skim milk is added for color to most varieties of commercially produced milk.

The next indignity is homogenization, the process of destroying the butter-fat found naturally in raw milk. Studies have shown that this process produces damaged fats that deposit onto the arterial walls contributing to the development of arteriosclerosis. Ronald Schmid, in his book, Traditional Foods Are Your Best Medicine (Healing Art Press, 1997), states that countries which do not homogenize their milk have heart disease rates less than half of that of the United States.

Modern processed milk puts an enormous strain on the body's systems. It is no wonder that so many people have adverse reactions to milk. We drink milk because we are told it will make our bodies healthy and stronger yet the vitamins, minerals, proteins, and fats that nature puts in raw milk from healthy cows is not available for absorption from devitalized pasteurized milk products. What our body does absorb are the toxic substances known to cause allergies, chronic fatigue, and a host of degenerative diseases.

What's a Girl to Do?

Unlike modern milk, organic raw or certified raw milk from pasture grazed cows is full of health building properties including fat-soluble vitamins, beneficial bacteria, and enzymes. One enzyme in particular, phosphatase, an element essential for calcium absorption, is rendered inactive from pasteurization. Fortified lifeless milk is no substitute for the health enhancing properties found in natural raw milk products from healthy animals.

11 Reasons
You and Your Family
Should Be Consuming Certified Raw Milk

- Raw milk contains essential amino acids
- Raw milk is a natural probiotic
- Raw milk is rich in antioxidants including B12
- Raw milk contains natural enzymes and fatty acids

Additionally, raw milk can help:

- strengthen the immune system
- lower cholesterol and triglycerides
- increase metabolic rate
- enhance muscle growth
- decrease abdominal fat
- lower insulin resistance
- reduce the severity or completely eliminate such conditions as: asthma, autism, osteoporosis, hypoglycemia, lactose intolerance, diabetes, and eczema.

You can read more about raw milk and find out where it can be purchased by going to www.realmilk.com or by contacting the Weston Price Foundation at www.westonaprice.org.

Question: Is the organic milk at the grocery store the same as raw milk?

Answer: No, not even close. Organic milk is both pasteurized and homogenized. And, like conventionally raise dairy cows, most are denied access to pasture. They live in concrete and steel environments on piles of manure, are artificially bred, and fed unnatural feed (grains). The result, a highly processed organic milk that is allergenic, has synthetic vitamins added to replace those lost during pasteurization, and can cause lactose intolerance since it is missing the beneficial enzymes found in raw milk. There are two things that separate organic pasteurized milk from conventional milk: one; USDA organic standards do not allow cows from organic dairies to be given hormones or antibiotics. And two; the grains fed to these cows must be organically grown. Grass by the way, is the natural diet for cows, not grains.

Please, do not let this confuse you. Yes, selecting organic products tends to always be a better choice over conventionally raised foods, except when it comes to milk and meat products. Remember, the organic label in these two instances only means that the cows were fed organic grains and not given antibiotics and steroids. Again, grains are NOT the natural diet of cows. And once the milk has been both pasteurized and homogenized, or even worse "ultra-pasteurized," its health-enhancing properties have been destroyed. You and your children deserve the highest quality milk and dairy products. Again, I encourage you to contact the Weston Price Foundation at Phone: (202) 363-4394, for assistance in locating real milk in your area.

The 7th Food
That Should Never Touch a Woman's Lips

Caffeine

Second to sugar, American's reach for their stimulant of choice, caffeine, through their favorite delivery systems...coffee, tea, and soft drinks. Nearly fifty percent of Americans drink, on average, three cups of coffee each day. The average cup of java contains about 75mg of caffeine while espresso sports about 100mg. Although tea leaves actually contain more caffeine than coffee beans, tea is generally prepared much weaker. And thanks to soda, America's children are getting hooked on caffeine (and sugar) at very early ages.

Caffeine is an alkaloid compound that stimulates the heart and the central nervous system, and is absorbed and distributed through the body rapidly. It is clearly one of the most highly used psychoactive substances used in the world. Classified as a stimulant type drug, the main function of caffeine is to alert body systems by stimulating the brain. Since it metabolizes rapidly, caffeine will reach all tissues within about five minutes. Maximum effects will be reached in about thirty minutes.

As few as one to two cups of coffee can produce a variety of physiological symptoms including increased pulse rate and increases in breathing and blood pressure. As two cups turn into three, four, then five, stronger side effects may be experienced such as: anxiety, rapid heart beat, insomnia, PMS (breast tenderness, irritability, and headaches), restlessness, and a disruption in sleep patterns. Other more serious side effects may include more frequent episodes of heartburn, mood and energy swings (as caffeine interferes with blood sugar levels resulting in a hypoglycemic reaction), irregular heart beat (cardiac arrhythmias), changes in bowel habits, conception related problems, and a possible increase in fibrocystic breast tissue.

The stimulating effects of caffeine leave the body in a constant state of emergency. Caffeine not only blocks the action of adenosine, the chemical in the brain that helps calm our nerves, it also stimulates the adrenal glands to produce the stress hormones adrenalin and cortisol in addition to more than 100 other hormones including testosterone and estrogen.

Our adrenal glands have similar characteristics to a bank savings account. Minor stress and the occasional double mocha cappuccino make minor withdrawals that are usually replenished quickly allowing us to remain in good health. Most women today however, make large frequent withdrawals from their adrenal reserves via nutritional and lifestyle factors that deplete their adrenal glands leaving them exhausted, and vulnerable to infections resulting from high cortisol levels and an overburdened immune system. Those with adrenal fatigue experience frequent sore throats, colds, and the flu.

What's a Girl to Do?

Ladies, I strongly encourage you to break the caffeine habit, as the long term effects can damage your health and most definitely drain your energy.

Author's note: For me, drinking coffee is what I refer to as, "Volunteering for my own misery." One cup of coffee will keep me awake all night, give me the shakes, drain my energy, result in a horrible migraine headache, and trigger the PMS of a very bad dream. And, if I really want to make myself feel horrible, all I need to do is consume something sweet or overly salty with a caffeinated beverage to make me feel like a monster has taken over my body; not very fun. Let's just say that when it comes to certain foods, I learned years ago to stop volunteering for my own misery.

The 8th Food
That Should Never Touch a Woman's Lips

Commercially Raised and Processed Meats

I would like to begin this section by stating that I am in no way advocating the exclusion of animal sources of protein in your diet (unless under the advice of your physician), as meat from healthy animals provides the body essential nutrients for growth and repair. The reason I have included commercially raised and processed meats as one of the 10 Foods is because meat from animals raised under the conditions I will describe below can pose potential short term and long term health consequences that you need to be aware of when purchasing meat for yourself and your family

The problem facing consumers of U.S. meat products is the pervasive contamination with antibiotics and steroid hormones that are passed on in every hamburger, steak, chop, rib, roast, wing, drum stick, boneless breast, hot dog, bratwurst, ham and Thanksgiving turkey.

Most modern livestock are housed in cramped quarters redolent with their own wastes, fed a diet specifically designed to fatten them up, and are allowed almost no interaction with the natural world around them. These conditions are ripe for a vast array of infectious diseases. Rather than being raised in a manner to promote health, the animals are given a host of antibiotics in order to suppress disease. These antibiotics eventually find their way into the food chain where they contribute to increasingly antibiotic resistant strains of bacteria in humans. The pharmaceutical industry must continually discover or create new antibiotics as the resistant stains become more prevalent.

26

To maximize profits, the animals are given hormones and steroids to induce larger-than-normal growth and milk production. For example, in the beef industry cows are fed synthetic hormones to accelerate growth, increase fat deposits, bring entire herds into heat at the same time for breeding, increase milk production, and induce abortions in pregnant cows scheduled for slaughter. These hormones are suspected as a major cause of the high incidence of breast and ovarian cancer in American women, as well as premature puberty in American children. Steroids are used to cause cattle to grow fat fast; it also stands to reason that they may in fact contribute to obesity in humans who consume the meat and milk of such contaminated animals.

Furthermore, US livestock also absorb all the herbicides, pesticides, and chemical fertilizers used to grow the feed crops on which they are forced to gorge and rarely, if ever, have access to their natural food source.

Commercially produced meats are also used to make most luncheon and deli-style meats including bacon, ham, bologna, sausage, pepperoni, hot dogs, jerky, and more. What makes these meat products poor food choices is not just the quality of the meat, but the ingredients added to them. The blue shimmer on the surface of luncheon meat is the result of sodium nitrate. Sodium nitrate is commonly used to keep meat looking red when it would have normally decomposed into an unappealing gray. In the stomach, sodium nitrate is converted into nitrous acid which is suspected of inciting cancers of the digestive tract. Additional chemical additives and preservatives are also used in processed meats including hydrolyzed protein, citric acid, spices, and natural flavors, MSG, sugar and large quantities of salt.

What's a Girl to Do?

In my home we eat meat and dairy products from cows that are pasture grazed (grass-fed). Grass-fed meats are rarely available in regular grocery stores, but can occasionally be found at specialty markets. Your best bet is to check the internet, and either order online, or locate a ranch near you and drive out to purchase your fresh meats directly from the farm. My husband and I drive forty-five minutes away to purchase our raw dairy products and grass-fed meat from a farmer who prides himself in caring for the land and his animals.

The following websites offer a wealth of valuable information on pasture grazed meats, including where to find stores, restaurants, Inns, and farms in your area that sell or serve food raised by farmers who practice traditional farming methods: www.eatwild.com, www.grasslandbeef.com, and www.eatwellguide.org.

Question: Are organic meats found at the grocery store the same as grass-fed meats?

Answer: No, most organic meats are from animals that were fed organically grown grains, and were not given synthetic hormones or antibiotics. This is certainly a better choice over commercially raised meats as described earlier in this section. However, grains are not the natural diet of these animals, which means that the nutrient balances in meats from grain-fed animals versus grass-fed (pasture grazed) animals will be different, specifically with regard to fatty acids.

The 9th and 10th Foods
That Should Never Touch a Woman's Lips

Processed and Fast Foods

There are more than 8,000 trade names and generic chemicals used worldwide in the manufacture and processing of foods. Food additives are used to enhance the texture, taste, and appearance of foods; to maintain or improve the overall nutritional quality of the food; and to extend the shelf life of the food.

The Standard American Diet is filled with processed foods wrapped in bright neon packages resembling the colors of fresh fruits and vegetables. Although the food industry has duped the public (with help from government health agencies) into believing that their products are safe for human consumption, there is abundant scientific evidence to the contrary. This information is in the public domain openly available to anyone who seeks it. Ignorance is therefore no longer a valid excuse for poisoning yourself with industrially adulterated foods.

The body correctly recognizes chemical food additives as toxic foreign agents and fights hard to remove them. Chemical food additives can cause severe biochemical reactions putting great stress on the immune system. After years of daily exposure to such inorganic chemicals the body becomes vulnerable to attack by microbes, toxins, and cancerous cells. If you have consumed such foods without noticeable damage to your health, it is the result of your body's strong resistance. The cumulative effects however, often unseen during youth, will increase with age as genetic weaknesses are uncovered which can lead to a host of degenerative diseases. When you stop poisoning cells, health improves.

29

Unfortunately, few women stop to consider that processed foods may negatively influence:

- Their ability to conceive
- The development of their baby in the womb
- The development of their growing children
- Their child's behavior
- Their inability to lose weight
- Their hormones
- Their emotional state
- Their energy levels
- Their ability to sleep through the night
- Their ability to wake up feeling refreshed
- Their ability to concentrate
- Their recovery when ill
- Their overall health and well-being
- Their ability to get through the day without additional stimulation from caffeine and sugar

38 Reasons to Not Eat Processed or Fast Food

Salt
Dextrose
Maltodextrin
Aspartame
Sucralose
Saccharin
Corn Syrup
High Fructose Corn
  Syrup
Partially Hydrogenated
  Oils (cottonseed oil,
  corn oil, soybean oil,
  palm kernel oil)
Carrageenan
Citric Acid
Butter Flavor
Sodium Citrate
Malic Acid
Blue #1
Red # 40
Caffeine
Fructose

Sodium Nitrate
Natural Flavor
Artificial Flavor
Enriched (synthetic
  vitamins)
Fortified (synthetic
  vitamins)
Monosodium Glutamate
Carmel Color
Acetylated Mono and
  Diglycerides BHA
  and BHT
Sodium Benzoate
Propylene Glycol
Yellow # 5 and # 6
Sodium Stearoyl
Polysorbate 60
Titanium Dioxide
Blue #2
Glycerin
Sorbitol
Emulsifiers

Inside Some Popular Processed Foods

Kellogg's® Special K Bars Peaches & Cream

rice
sugar
whole grain wheat
wheat gluten
defatted wheat germ
salt
wheat flour
malt flavoring
maltodextrin
riboflavin
thiamin hydrochloride
corn syrup
fructose
partially hydrogenated
soybean, cottonseed, and
palm kernel oils
dextrose
dried peach
golden raisins

glycerine
annatto
sodium bisulfite
strawberry flavored fruit pieces
cranberries
citric acid
elderberry juice
non-fat dry milk
sorbitol
natural and artificial strawberry
and peach flavors
soy lecithin
calcium carbonate
natural yogurt flavor
niacinamide
artificial flavor
BHT
pyridoxine hydrochloride

Atkins™ Endulge Ice cream

cream
nonfat dry milk
whey
sorbitol
polydextrose
guar gum
mono & diglycerides

xanthan gum
polysorbate 80
carrageenan
natural and artificial vanilla
flavor
sucralose* Splenda®

Frito Lay Crunchy Cheetos®

enriched corn meal
vegetable oil
whey
salt
cheddar cheese
partially hydrogenated
soybean oil
maltodextrin,

modified food starch
 disodium phosphate
sour cream
artificial flavor
MSG
lactic acid
yellow #6
citric acid

Diet Coke®

carbonated water
caramel color
phosphoric acid
sodium saccharin
potassium benzoate (to
protect taste)
natural flavors
citric acid

caffeine
potassium citrate
aspartame: aspartame
contains phenylalanine
dimethylpolysiloxane
Phenylketonurics:
contains phenylalanine

Jello® Sugar Free-Fat Free Instant
White Chocolate Artificial Flavor

modified food starch
maltodextrin
tetrasodium
pyrpphosphate
and
disodium phosphate
contains less than 2% of
skim milk
natural and artificial
flavor

salt
calcium sulfate
xanthan gum
mono and diglycerides
aspartame
acesulfame potassium
yellow 5

Jolly Time® Healthy Pop Kettle Corn Microwave Popcorn

pop corn
partially hydrogenated soybean oil
salt
modified food starch
sucralose
artificial flavor
soy lecithin
annatto

Atkins™ Chocolate and Coconut Bar

soy protein
hydrolyzed collagen
whey protein
calcium/sodium caseinate
glycerin
polydextrose
water
cocoa butter
natural coconut oil
coconut
cellulose
cocoa powder
olive oil
lecithin
natural and artificial
flavor
maltodextrin
guar gum
citric acid
sucralose (Splenda®)

tricalcium phosphate
calcium carbonate
magnesium oxide
vitamin A
vitamin C
thiamin (B$_1$)
riboflavin (B$_2$)
pyridoxide (B$_6$)
cyanocobalamin (B$_{12}$)
natural vitamin E
(Acetate)
niacin
biotin
pantothenic acid
zinc
folic acid
chromium chelate
vitamin K
selenium

Crystal Light® Lemonade

citric acid
potassium citrate
aspartame: contains
Phenylalanine
magnesium oxide

lemon juice solids
acesulfame potassium
artificial color
yellow 5 lake
BHA

Slim Fast® Optima:
45% less-sugar Milk Chocolate Flavor

maltodextrin
sugar
cocoa
high oleic sunflower oil
gum arabic
cellulose gel
milk protein concentrate
buttermilk powder
soybean lecithin
xanthan gum
dextrose
carrageenan,
modified corn starch
salt
potassium phosphate
acesulfame potassium
cyanocobalamin &
cholecalciferol
aspartame

artificial Flavor
guar gum
corn starch
ferric orthophosphate
zinc, niacin,
calcium pantothenenate
manganese sulfate
pyridoxide hydrochloride
thiamine mononitrate
vitamin A palmitate
chromium chloride
riboflavin, folic acid
copper gluconate
sodium molybdate
sodium selenite, biotin
potassium iodide
phytonadione

Fruit by the Foot®

grapes from concentrate
sugar
maltodextrin
corn syrup
pear concentrate
partially hydrogenated
cottonseed oil
carrageenan
citric acid
distilled monoglycerides
sodium citrate

malic acid
acetylated mono and
diglycerides
xanthum gum
vitamin C
locust bean gum
potassium citrate
red #40
natural and artificial
flavor

Kraft® Fat-Free™ Thousand Island Dressing

tomato puree
high fructose corn syrup
water
chopped pickles
modified food starch
maltodextrin
soybean oil
egg yolks
xanthan gum
artificial color
mustard flour
potassium sorbate

calcium sodium EDTA,
phosphoric acid
dried onions
guar gum
spice
vitamin E
lemon juice concentrate
yellow 6
natural flavor
red 40
artificial flavor
blue 1

Crisco®

partially hydrogenated soybean and cottonseed oils
mono and diglycerides

Sugar-Free SnackWell's ®Fudge Brownie Cookies

enriched bleach flour
(niacin, reduced iron,
thiamine mononitrate,
riboflavin, folic acid)
maltitol
hydrogenated glucose
syrup
partially hydrogenated
soybean and cottonseed
oil
sorbitol
cocoa (processed with
alkali)
egg whites
chocolate
water
emulsifiers
vegetable mono and
diglycerides

soy lecithin
propylene glycol
mono-and diesters of
fatty acids
baking soda
salt, glycerin
modified food starch
polydextrose
maltodextrin
sodium alginate
yellow corn flour
malic acid
artificial flavor
sucralose
camel color
milk

Wheat Thins® Baked Snack Crackers

enriched flour
(niacin, reduced iron,
thiamin mononitrate,
riboflavin, folic acid)
partially hydrogenated
soybean oil
defatted wheat germ
sugar
corn starch
high fructose corn syrup
salt
corn syrup

monoglycerides
malt syrup
leavening
artificial color

McDonald's Strawberry Triple Thick® Shake

whole milk
sucrose
cream, nonfat milk solids
corn syrup solids
mono and diglycerides
guar gum
imitation vanilla flavor
carrageenan
cellulose gum
vitamin A palmitate

Strawberry Syrup: sugar
strawberries
water,
high fructose corn syrup
corn syrup
natural (vegetable source) and artificial flavor
pectin
citric acid
xanthan gum
potassium sorbate (a preservative)
caramel color
FD&C red #40
calcium chloride
May contain small amounts of other shake flavors served at
the restaurant, including egg ingredients when
Egg Nog Shakes are available.

Chapter 2

The Toxic Cloud of Dietary Confusion

In this chapter I will be addressing what I refer to as "The Toxic Cloud of Dietary Confusion" surrounding modern nutrition. Today's ever changing and always conflicting dietary directives are leaving women either indifferent to their nutritional needs or constantly pursuing a nutritious eating plan they can fit into their busy schedules. Unfortunately, as their constantly shifting eating plans fail to yield the desired results, many women find themselves moving even farther away from their goals as they wander through the following clouds of dietary confusion.

Categories of Dietary Confusion

I'm Desperate to Lose Weight; I'll Do Anything Except...

When women seek my services, it never fails to amaze me how similar each consultation is to the next; how often I hear the same refrain. "Dr. Doll, I'm here to lose weight. I'm desperate; I'll do whatever you say. I've been on every diet out there, I've even tried exercising but nothing works. My body is resistant to losing weight." Interestingly, during the initial consultation, few women mention their health problems. If they do bring them up they diminish their relevance well below the ever-present need to lose weight. I have yet to counsel anyone who has sought my services in their valiant pursuit of vibrant health and longevity; on the contrary...it's all about the weight loss.

Now don't get me wrong, desiring to lose weight is certainly a worthy goal since waistlines across America resemble that of the Michelin man. And, if in losing weight some of their health problems diminish, most women would certainly be happy. However, it has been both my personal and my professional experience, that for most women it's all about the weight loss, weight loss at any cost: low carb, high protein, low fat, the right fat, fasting, surgeries, low calorie, the banana diet, the grapefruit diet, Dr. So and So's Diet, national strip-mall diets, celebrity diets, doctor supervised diets; and of course, Joe Bob's diet soda and deli sandwich diet. The list could fill volumes.

My opinion about all of these weight loss marketing plans can be summed up in two words: brilliant and insane. These products are brilliant, if you are the marketing genius behind these multi-billion dollar money makers. They are insane if you are the woman futilely doing the same thing over and over and expecting a different result.

In truth, most women come to me seeking the same sales pitch. They want me to tell them that they can lose weight and get in shape without giving up their favorite foods and with minimal exercise. Translated, "I am unwilling to give up junk food and I hate to exercise. Therefore, unless you can tell me how I can look like you without adopting your eating and lifestyle habits I will quietly miss my next appointment and move on. I will continue seeking out the *expert* or *program* that promises me a diet of soda and scones, along with the occasional stroll to my mailbox will result in a lean, fit, healthy body."

Ladies, when it comes to being healthy and fit, there are no short cuts. And until you stop paying the carnival magician for his bag of tricks, your anger and frustration will only increase, right along with your weight and health problems.

The Similarities Between Diets and Abusive Relationships

- They offer promises they can't keep.
- They rob you of your dignity.
- They lack a genuine concern for your needs.
- They try and convince you that potentially dangerous (behaviors/foods/programs) are really good for you.
- They offer gifts to reel you in.
- They drain your energy (vitality).
- They have unreasonable expectations.
- They interfere with your sleep.
- You keep going back to them because they assure you that things will be different this time, you won't make the same mistakes.
- You loose your ability to recognize what healthy foods or a healthy relationship with food looks like.
- We defend them, and then blame ourselves for our failure.
- They can seriously damage your health or even kill you.

All Foods are Part of a Healthy Diet

I have never really been sure if those who argue with me that all foods are part of a healthy diet really believe it. Yes, a wide variety of whole-foods are part of a healthy diet. However, faux-foods which are chemically filled, artificially flavored, colored, and preserved, are NOT part of a healthy diet.

Now, if you choose to consume these embalmed foods on occasion, hopefully you do so only if you are in excellent health. Most healthy people can handle the occasional intrusion of processed foods into their diet

41

without experiencing any short or long-term ill effects. However, if you are chronically ill, overweight, trying to get pregnant, pregnant, nursing, or over age 60, I strongly advise you to avoid the 10 foods listed in Chapter 1. Salt, white flour and sugar, artificial sweeteners, pasteurized milk, damaged fats, caffeinated beverages, commercially raised and processed meats, along with processed and fast foods, interfere with the body's ability to heal itself, maintain a healthy immune system, lose weight, or conceive and have a healthy pregnancy.

Diet Withdrawals

Most women are unaware of the addictive nature of processed foods. Like other addicting substances, they offer a temporary high followed by the inevitable crash. Any attempt to go off of them abruptly almost always results in withdrawal symptoms.

For example, artificial sweeteners, caffeine, and hydrogenated oils, refined sugars, along with foods containing artificial flavors and colors, flood our brain's receptors with chemical stimulants. Having grown accustomed to this stimulation through frequent ingestion of processed foods, women often experience classic symptoms of chemical withdrawals when these foods are removed from the diet. Anyone who has ever tried to quit drinking coffee will attest to this. Similar reactions can result when large quantities of white flour and sugar are suddenly removed from the diet: headaches, irritability, foggy thinking, drowsiness, anxiety, and so forth. Symptoms fade when the foods are returned to the body or after the body has adjusted to their absence. This is why women frequently tell me that they feel more energetic when they eat junk foods and that fresh foods do not give them the same surges of energy; what they are feeling is not really a surge of energy, it is relief from withdrawals.

Unfortunately, as with other addictive substances, the brain builds up a tolerance to the chemical stimulants found in processed foods. Over time it will demand more and more of these chemicals to keep us going and feeling satisfied or "normal." Our bodies however, can only take this chemical abuse for so long and will eventually become ill. When this revolt occurs and how it manifests itself within the body will vary from person to person.

Ladies, if this describes you, please understand that continuing to eat foods that artificially stimulate your system will only serve to interfere with any attempts you make to improve your health. Eat real food!

Conflicting Dietary Advice

This next group of women I'd like to discuss may be very familiar to most of you. In fact, you might be one of the millions of women lost in the cloud of conflicting dietary advice. Those in this category may or may not need to lose weight per se; they are simply trying to feed themselves and their families' healthy meals. Where do they get their dietary advice? Generally from a number of sources: the government, their doctor, a nutrition professional, the Heart Association, books, television, school, etc. Whatever the source, there is one thing they can be sure of...conflicting advice.

Ladies, the only foods you need to worry about, as I will discuss in Chapter 4, are the ones you can in essence hunt, gather, fish, pick from a tree, or raise on a farm; foods consumed as close to their natural state as possible. You do not need to worry about high protein, low-fat, low carb, counting calories, or any of the other diet fads that come along including the ancillary snake oil products that accompany them. What do I mean by snake oil products?

- **Frozen Diet Foods**
  Frequently high in salt in addition to artificial sweeteners, flavors, colors, preservatives, and hydrogenated oils

- **Meal Replacement Shakes and Bars**
  The ingredients alone should be enough to prevent you from letting these faux foods touch your lips. Note examples in Chapter 1.

- **Sports or Energy Bars**
  Numerous refined and artificial sugars, synthetic vitamins, artificial flavors, partially hydrogenated oils, and preservatives

- **Low-Carb Cakes, Cookies,**
  Pancake Mixes, Chips, Bread, etc
  Funny how the high protein gurus tell you not to eat carbs then turn around and manufacture a full array of processed carbs they tell you are "OK" to eat. These faux foods are simply artificially flavored, colored, sweetened and embalmed replacement carbohydrates. Just eat real food!

- **Low-Fat This and Sugar-Free That**
  Lite or Lean It's all the Same
  Translated: Take out something good; add in something bad. Or, take out something bad and add in something worse. I repeat...eat real food.

What's all of the Fuss About?

This cloud of dietary confusion surrounds far too many of our nation's senior citizens. They were the first generation to grow up and come of age with television, TV dinners, canned and packaged foods, and products such as Crisco®. They were the teenagers that helped launch hamburger
chains. This generation came of age when these products were exciting and new. We must also note that they were also children during periods in our nation's history when food was often scarce. Hence, they grew up being told to eat what was in front of them and to be grateful for what food they had.

Sadly, as the people in this age group begin to experience health problems associated with years of eating damaged fats (Crisco® and margarine), table salt, canned and processed foods, along with pasteurized dairy products, they rarely consider that these foods might be contributing to their heart disease, high blood pressure, osteoporosis, cancer, diabetes, and weight issues. After all, they have been convinced by many of their healthcare providers and marketed by pharmaceutical manufactures that these conditions are "just a part of aging." Rarely do today's health professionals recognize or admit that America's health crisis has in fact been spawned from years of consuming lifeless foods.

My heart goes out to those in this generation because they have been effectively conditioned to believe that many of these nutrient-deplete foods are good for them, or at least not bad. Because of their age, seniors require the highest quality foods to support a strong immune system. Instead, far too many in this age group are living on a diet of fruit-cocktail, instant cereals, white bread and sugar, canned corn and instant mashed potatoes smothered in margarine.

If you disagree with me, I invite you to make a visit to the nearest senior citizen's care facility.

Is Nutrition That Difficult to Understand?

Eating is an instinctive process. We are hard wired to seek out foods to nourish, strengthen, and heal our bodies. For millions of years man has hunted and gathered his food from the land without thought to its calorie, fat, or carbohydrate content. Today, things are very different. Consumers have been slickly marketed into believing that nutrition is too difficult to understand, and that processed foods are equal to, if not better for them than real foods. Conflicting dietary advice, over-burdened schedules, and the ever-increasing presence of fast and convenience food have resulted in a nation that is obese, exhausted, chronically ill, and confused about nutrition. Is nutrition really that difficult to understand, or are we simply being conditioned to choose fake foods over real foods?

I illustrated this point in a recent newsletter I wrote for my website www.cristidoll.com.

Ideas for Healthy Living Newsletter
April 2006

By: Cristi J. Doll, Ph.D.

Are Americans Afraid to Eat Real Food?

Those who peddle processed foods have done a marvelous job convincing Americans that the ever rising number of meal replacement shakes, bars, and prepackaged meals are equivalent, if not better for them than real foods, and far more convenient. Unfortunately, many of those we trust to have our best interest in mind such as our fitness and health care professionals, frequently lead the pack when it comes recommending these products as substitutes for regular meals. Here is an example.

As I walked into the gym the other morning, one of the trainers was doing his best to convince a middle-aged couple that they needed to invest in their health by investing in some meal replacement powders, bars, and assorted supplements. I listened as he praised the health and fat-burning virtues of these products. The man and woman, each approximately 45 years old and 30lbs to 40lbs overweight, expressed how they were beginning to experience health related issues resulting from years of poor food choices and lack of physical activity. They also stated that they were confused by all of the contradictions surrounding nutrition and that they were too tired in the evenings to prepare meals.

It was only a matter of minutes before these folks had signed up to receive the gym's complete monthly weight loss package consisting of: 28 meal replacement bars, 28 servings of meal replacement shake mix, your very own shaker bottle, and 1 bottle of fat burning complex, all designed to take the guess work and stress out of meal time. (* The package also included some personal training sessions and some nutrition counseling). The trainer went on to emphasize the nutritional value of these products, and how they were key components to achieving their weight loss and fitness goals. In other words, these folks were being conditioned to believe that their success hinged on the inclusion of these meal "replacement" foods and fat-burning supplements. Also stressed was their need to continue purchasing these products even after they reached their weight loss goals, to help them maintain their results.

Here is another example; I had a woman come to me for help with losing 25lbs before she became pregnant. She said she had tried every diet out there but nothing worked. Upon review of her health questionnaire and two-week food diary, I quickly discovered that this 32 year old woman had had three miscarriages in the past two years, and was suffering with chronic fatigue, neither of which she mentioned during our interview. Her diet consisted primarily of meal replacement shakes that her doctor had recommended to help her lose weight.

After reviewing the meal plan I had written for her, she gasped and replied, "I can't eat these foods; they'll make me fat." When I asked if she had ever considered that her diet might be a contributing factor with her inability to conceive or her chronic fatigue she said, "No, I believe these foods are the reason I haven't gained any more weight, and that once I lose this weight, I will be less likely to miscarry or be tired." Sadly, she was unwilling to follow the food suggestions I had given her for fear of gaining more weight, and did not want to hear that the large amount of pseudo foods she was eating might be the cause of her problems. Like so many other women, she had been conditioned to fear real food. While it is certainly true that miscarriages and chronic fatigue can result from carrying excess weight, in her case, one could easily include that her poor nutrition was a strong contributing factor in each of these conditions.

When a 50 year old woman tells me that her excess weight and health challenges are the result of eating too many almonds and pecans, I know she has been conditioned to fear real food. When a 40 year old woman tells me she cannot include sliced avocado on her salad at lunch because it will contribute to middle-age spread, she too has been conditioned to fear real food. And when a 32 year old woman conceives, after she and her husband remove all processed foods from their diet for six months, they learn to embrace rather than fear real foods after battling infertility for over five years.

Now I will pose the question to you, "Are you one of the millions of Americans who has been conditioned to fear real food?"

What's a Girl to Do?

The next time you sit down to a frozen weight loss meal, diet soda, rice cake, low-fat bagel, or a meal replacement drink or bar, ask yourself the following questions, "Are these imitation foods going to improve my health and help me to achieve the lean, energetic body I desire? Or, are these foods contributing to my health problems, draining my energy, and interfering with my ability to lose weight?" Then ask yourself if nutrition is really that difficult to understand.

Chapter 3

I Would Love to Eat Right But...

I don't like vegetables.
Healthy foods taste bad.
I still gain weight.
Healthy foods are too expensive.
There's no time to cook.
I hate to cook.
My family won't eat healthy foods.
Pretzels, chocolates, and diet sodas are my only vice.
I take vitamins.
I eat salad sometimes.
I know how to eat right I just don't do it.
I only buy the goodies for my kids.
I am unwilling to give up _____, _____, and _____.
I eat low-fat foods.
I eat right most of the time.
I'm on _____ Diet.
A few Twinkies now and then never hurt anyone.
Organic foods are difficult to locate.

In this chapter, I will be responding to some of the top reasons women have given me over the years for not eating right.

"I would love to eat healthy food but I just don't have TIME to prepare it."

The single greatest reason women cite for not eating right (or exercising) is lack of time. Since proper nutrition is essential to good health, shopping for and preparing nutritious meals must be scheduled into our lives with priority status just like anything else in our lives we value. Sadly, millions of women devalue this natural health enhancer as evidenced by their poor eating habits, their expanding waistlines, and the rise in chronic illness.

One of the most direct choices we make every day is what to put in our mouths. Eating should be relaxing and enjoyable; instead, eating has become complicated and disruptive. Because of the fast pace of modern life, eating is more often an exercise in refueling than a festivity. Most people tell themselves that healthy foods cost too much and take too long to prepare. In the end we must ask ourselves if the time we save microwaving a frozen dinner, opening a can of soup, or stopping off for cheap burger combos, have in fact saved us money and afforded more time to: read with our children, take a walk with our spouse, take an art class, or find a quite place to unwind and reflect? Most of us will agree that such eating practices have only served to frazzle our nerves, have contributed to our fatigue and health problems, and have certainly interfered with valuable time we could have spent preparing and enjoying delicious, nutritious, and pleasurable meals with those we love.

"I have inherited fat genes."

Women frequently tell me they have inherited fat genes or have a slow metabolism. Genetics do of course play a significant role in determining our body type and whether we are pre-disposed to certain health conditions, including the body's ability to gain weight and store fat. A predisposition however, does not mean that you will become sick or fat. Yes, genetics strongly influence why some women can eat anything and everything without gaining weight or becoming ill, while others seem to gain weight and get yeast infections just thinking about cake. A slow metabolism however, is the result of muscle loss and unstable blood sugar; and a lack of muscle tissue is directly related to insufficient physical activity and inadequate nutrition.

Obesity is not a trait like eye color, which is determined at the moment of conception; it is a tendency for obesity that is inherited. Obesity needs to have an environment that will nurture its development before it becomes a reality. Eating nutrient dense foods and participating in a progressive fitness program is essential for women born with the genetic tendency to store fat easily.

"Eating a Few Twinkies Now and Then Never Hurt Anyone"

Ok, you're right, eating a Twinkie now and then probably won't kill you, nor will siphoning gasoline out of your car from time to time; nevertheless, I do not recommend either one. I am always amazed at how many women will actually pay for my services then argue with me over this point. Ladies, it's not the occasional Twinkie, donut, handful of chips, or skipped workout that damages your health, drains your energy, and prevents you from getting into shape. It's the twenty plus years of skipped workouts, Twinkies, donuts, candy bars, fast-food meals, coffee beverages, diet sodas, and bags of chips that can lead to heart disease, obesity, and cancer and make you feel like garbage along the way.

There really are no excuses to put health depleting foods into our mouths when there are so many delicious alternatives. Fabulous and nutritious desserts and snacks can be made from fresh ingredients or purchased from specialty stores or bakeries such as Whole Foods or online from Diamond Organics.

"I only buy the goodies for my kids."

When women tell me that they only buy the goodies for the kids, I look them straight in the eyes and ask, "Ok, let me get this straight, are you telling me that none of these foods wind up in your purse or your desk drawers at work?" If this sounds a little bit too familiar, then you might want to brace yourself when you hear me say, "Stop buying junk food; stop hiding it in your purse or desk drawers, stop eating at fast food restaurants, and stop using your kids as your reason for buying these foods in the first place." You and your family need to be eating real foods.

Meet Janet

Janet does not exercise or eat right. She is 43 years old, 40 lbs overweight, and the mother of two. Both of her children were conceived with the help of fertility drugs following three miscarriages in five years. Janet also has high blood pressure, diabetes, and debilitating PMS.

Janet can't remember the last time she exercised or even felt good. She drags out of bed most mornings after sleeping through her alarm. She and her husband stumble to get to the coffee pot and to light their cigarettes. Cold, sugar-coated cereal is breakfast on most mornings or they grab something from a drive-thru window on their way to work and school. If Janet does pack lunches for her children they generally consist of bologna on white bread, fruit roll-ups, chips, candy, and a can of soda. Her husband eats from the catering truck while Janet and the girls from the office drive down to the mall to lunch at the food court.

By 3pm Janet's energy has crashed and her head is pounding. She reaches into her desk for a candy bar and pops open her fourth can of soda to give her the lift she needs to get through her day until she picks up the kids. On the way to baseball practice they will blow through their favorite drive-thru window for dinner. During ball practice Janet sits with the other mothers in lawn chairs drinking diet sodas and eating chips and M&Ms. By the time she gets home her nerves are shot and she has a full-blown migraine. She reaches for her nightly anxiety pill and pain reliever.

On the nights when Janet does prepare dinner for her family it usually starts from something frozen like pizza, or from a box or can like macaroni and cheese or canned spaghetti. After dinner they sit in front of the TV drinking sodas and eating a buffet of processed snack foods. Over the course of a single week Janet consumes on average twenty diet sodas, four to seven bowls of sugary cereal, nine candy bars, a large bag of chips, five donuts, six fast food meals, and does not exercise.

Although Janet hates the way she feels and would like to lose some weight, every diet she has ever tried has failed and she loathes exercise. To complicate matters more, all suggestions to improve her family's eating habits are met with stern objections. Her husband becomes particularly defensive as he sees nothing wrong with the way they eat. Even when the family budget is tight, Janet's husband refuses to stop spending money on his favorite foods and insists they cut expenses elsewhere. He frequently retorts, "There is nothing wrong with the way this family eats. Besides, it is perfectly natural for adults to gain weight as they age."

Janet's family is clearly lost in a toxic cloud of food chemicals, weight-loss, dietary confusion, and excuses.

Chapter 4

Coming Out of the Clouds:
Learning to Recognize Real Foods

Nutrition Should Be About Good Health
Not Just Weight Loss

When I counsel women about nutrition and exercise I let them know that before they can make internal and external changes in their bodies they must first acknowledge that a vibrant, energetic, and fit body is the result of healthy lifestyle habits that carry over year after year throughout the seasons of their lives. Until they have a desire for good health and not simply an obsession with weight loss, their health challenges will likely continue.

Proper nutrients lay the foundation for good health. A healthy eating plan provides the body its nutritional needs consistently from childhood through our senior years. Adjustments will be made in the quantity of food consumed only, as fuel needs will vary to meet specific demands placed on the body such as growth, pregnancy, physical activity (workload), or illness. No changes should occur in the foods themselves and quality should remain consistent.

Ladies, the foods necessary to support good health have not changed for thousands of years yet few people today recognize *real* food, how it is supposed to look and taste, where it comes from, or how it should be raised. This is evidenced by the fact that the preferred diet of America's women (and men) contains mostly foods from Chapter 1 in this book, processed and nutrient-deplete, health draining instead of health building. These terms describe not only the foods themselves, but the way these cheap calories are grown to create low quality foods.

Deciding Where to Hunt and Gather

Real foods, as opposed to processed foods, are foods that one could in essence hunt, gather, or fish for in the wild. Foods like the ones our great grandparents and those before them used as both nourishment and medicine. Foods our cells need to build healthy immune systems, lean strong bodies, and create sustained energy.

Unfortunately, some of the healthiest foods are not available in stores; they must be purchased directly from the farm, a farmer's market, a co-op, or a specialty store such as Whole Foods Market. Earlier, I stated that in our home we eat only grass-fed meats, raw dairy products, and either organically grown produce, or produce grown by farmers who practice traditional farming methods. Since moving to Philadelphia, my husband and I drive forty-five minutes away to stock up on delicious raw dairy products and grass-fed meats from Hendricks Farms and Dairy in Telford, Pennsylvania. Each month, Hendrick's Farms has over 1,000 families who drive from five different states to purchase farm fresh food from healthy animals. If we are unable to make the trip out to the farm, Hendricks raw milk and award winning cheeses are available locally from the market at Shady Brook Farm in Yardley Pennsylvania, and we order our grass-fed meat online from US Wellness meats: www.grasslandbeef.com.

In addition to our own backyard garden, we also belong to an organic fruit and vegetable cooperative farm. During the growing season we spend our Saturday mornings driving about 20 minutes away to Pennington, New Jersey to pick up our share of freshly picked organic fruits, vegetables, and herbs from Honey Brook Organic Farm.

Many neighborhoods throughout the country have community supported agriculture, where groups of people come together to support local farmers who practice traditional methods of farming. The following websites will give you more information about traditional farming practices and will help you locate such a farm, ranch, co-op, or certified farmer's market near you.

- www.westonaprice.org
- www.eatwild.com
- www.grasslandbeef.com
- www.realmilk.com
- www.cafarmersmarkets.com
- www.eatwellguide.org
- www.organicconsumers.org
- www.ams.usda.gov/farmersmarkets/map.htm
- www.biodynamics.com/csa.html

What Does "Organic" Mean?

Most of you have probably heard the term "organic" in reference to fruits and vegetables. Did you know that this term also applies to meat, eggs, dairy products, nuts, and whole-grains? Understanding the difference between organic and conventionally raised foods will help you make the best choices for you and your family.

The U.S. Government's Definition of Organic

What is organic food?

Organic food is produced by farmers who emphasize the use of renewable resources and the conservation of soil and water to enhance environmental quality for future generations. Organic meat, poultry, eggs, and dairy products come from animals that are given no antibiotics or growth hormones. Organic food is produced without using most conventional pesticides; fertilizers made with synthetic ingredients or sewage sludge; bioengineering; or ionizing radiation. Before a product can be labeled "organic," a Government-approved certifier inspects the farm where the food is grown to make sure the farmer is following all the rules necessary to meet USDA organic standards. Companies that handle or process organic food before it gets to your local supermarket or restaurant must be certified, too.

Is organic food better for me and my family?

USDA makes no claims that organically produced food is safer or more nutritious than conventionally produced food. Organic food differs from conventionally produced food in the way it is grown, handled, and processed.

When I go to the supermarket, how can I tell organically produced food from conventionally produced food?

You must look at package labels and watch for signs in the supermarket. Along with the national organic standards, USDA developed strict labeling rules to help consumers know the exact organic content of the food they buy. The USDA Organic seal also tells you that a product is at least 95 percent organic.

Does *natural* mean *organic*?

No. Natural and organic are not interchangeable. Other truthful claims, such as free-range, hormone-free, and natural, can still appear on food labels. However, don't confuse these terms with "organic." Only food labeled "organic" has been certified as meeting USDA organic standards.

Excerpted from:
www.ams.usda.gov/nop/Consumers/brochure.html
For more detailed information on the USDA organic standards, visit our web site at
http://www.ams.usda.gov/nop call the National Organic Program at 202-720-3252, or write USDA-AMS-TM-NOP, Room 4008 S. Bldg., Ag Stop 0268, 1400 Independence, SW, Washington, DC 20250.

Should You Choose Organic?

Many people ask me if organic foods are better for their health than conventionally raised foods. In a perfect world, all foods would be raised and processed in a fashion that is conducive to the health and well-being of the animal, the plant, the soil, the environment, and of course...the consumer. Since this is clearly not the case, it is up to the individual to decide what is best for his or her specific needs. Those who make the decision to buy organic usually do so because they prefer to consume foods that have not been genetically modified, and have been spared the application of dangerous chemicals (synthetic fertilizers, pesticides, growth hormones, antibiotics, etc.). These consumers also prefer foods that have been grown or raised in a fashion that is more humane and environmentally conscious for both animals and the land.

Organic foods are NOT always the healthiest as we learned earlier; specifically in reference to meats and dairy products. Yes, it is no wonder consumers are confused. Just be careful when selecting meat and dairy products to help ensure that you and your family are receiving the highest quality food available. It is worth your time to familiarize yourself with the websites listed earlier in this section.

Words of Wisdom

- If it has been pasteurized, chemically preserved, bleached, hydrogenated, salted, artificially colored, highly sugared, de-fibered, sterilized, canned, artificially sweetened, synthetically fortified, or filled with chemicals, do no eat it!

- The multi-billion dollar processed food industry would like you to believe their foods are "part of a healthy diet." It's a lie!

- Our bodies are designed to thrive on foods that are as close to the way nature provides them as possible.

- You can not make up for years of poor food choices by taking synthetic vitamins. Eat the real food source!

- Steer clear of any diet or nutrition program that includes chemically filled, artificially flavored, synthetically fortified processed food as part of a healthy, balanced diet; this includes meal replacement bars or drinks, and frozen "diet" foods/meals.

- Only you control what goes into your mouth.

- Low-fat diets can lead to hormone imbalance, a flabby body, cravings for sugar and stimulants, brittle nails and hair, insomnia, extreme fatigue, and mood swings, and problems conceiving.

- For those of you who make the excuse that organic products are too expensive, so are medical bills and junk food.

- It is just as easy to grab an apple as it is a package of potato chips.

- Plant a vegetable garden. It's easy, very inexpensive, a stress buster, and great exercise. Vegetables can thrive in the smallest of areas, even in pots. Find a neighbor who has experience growing vegetables in your area to help you get started. Gardeners love sharing their knowledge with others.

- If you are ill, over age sixty, attempting to become pregnant, pregnant, or nursing, you cannot afford to eat devitalized foods.

- Plan ahead, prepared ahead; I cannot say this enough.

Higher Quality Prepackaged Foods

I know that some of you are saying to yourself right now, "Alright, I am willing to do what it takes to acquire fresh produce. I do not even mind driving a ways if necessary to obtain grass-fed meat and raw dairy products. I am even willing to prepare the majority of my family's meals. However, I do not have the time, the expertise, or the resources to make spaghetti sauce, peanut butter, breads, and so forth." Not to worry my friends; thankfully, there are many companies that produce a variety of high-quality, chemical free organic foods including pastas, sauces, juices, soups, cookies, deli-meats, cereals, and raw nut butters. Here are some of my favorites.

- Bob's Red Mill: grains, flours, and cereals: www.bobsredmill.com

- Seeds of Change, produces some of my favorite products. They insist on quality, which you will clearly taste when you try their foods. Their sauces, dressings, and salsas are a regular part of our meals. Visit www.seedsofchange.com where you will find great ideas for organic eating and living.

- Muir Glenn organic sauces are in a word, (fabulous). Their products are available at many mainstream and natural food stores.

- Walnut Acres: Their slogan is, "Live pure." Once you taste their soups, salsas, sauces, and juices, you will know why. Visit www.walnutacres.com.

- Nature's Path Organic Manna Bread (I honestly do not know how I could get through life without this bread). Visit www.naturespath.com for a list of all of their delicious foods which are available from many mainstream grocers as well as natural food stores.

- Spectrum Naturals has a variety of expeller-pressed oils, dressings, and more.

- Garden of Eatin. I get hungry just visiting their site, www.gardenofeatin.com. My family loves foods from this company which can now be found in many mainstream grocery stores in addition to natural food stores.

- Pacific Organic Soups (I use their broths for all of my soup bases). Get the low or no salt versions. www.pacificfoods.com. Their soups are delicious, and they make cooking a breeze.

- Maranatha nut butters: www.nspriredfoods.com

- Sea Salt: www.realsalt.com

- Organic chocolate: An internet search will help you locate a variety of quality organic chocolates. I frequently use Sunspire® Natural Chocolates.

- Omega Nutrition: 100% Organic Coconut Oil www.omeganutrition.com

- Hodgson ® Mill: grains. www.hodgsonmill.com. I use these grains for my cooking needs daily.

- Frontier™ Culinary Spices. Available at many mainstream grocers and natural food stores.

Meet Lori

Lori is 36 years old and the mother of three. Lori weighs 120 lbs, and eats mostly organic foods. Exercise is a priority for Lori and her lifestyle reflects this. Lori gets up at 5:30 AM to get in a bike ride or to do calisthenics on the back porch. She stops to pick vegetables from her garden before heading into the house. By 6:30 she is fixing breakfast and packing healthy lunches for herself, her husband, and the kids.

Lori's family has many favorite breakfast and lunch foods including: omelets, homemade granola or muffins, fresh fruit, nitrate-free bacon, waffles, grilled chicken sandwiches, oatmeal cookies, raw vegetables, chili, and raw nuts. Lori prepares many of these foods over the weekend to make busy weekday meals quick and nutritious.

While at work, Lori grazes all day on the food she brings from home. During her lunch hour she can be found sitting out under a tree eating and reading a book, or meeting her husband or best-friend for a walk in the park. On nights when the kids have soccer practice, Lori packs an ice-chest the night before and keeps it in her car trunk while she is at work; no rushing, no drive-thru windows, great food. During practice she can be found walking or jogging around the fields. On the weekends Lori looks after her garden, rollerblades with her kids, mountain bikes and attends baseball games with her husband, and prepares much of the week's food ahead of time. She is happy and her lifestyle and health reflect her personality and priorities.

Lori and families like hers are rapidly being crowded out by families like Janet's as the epidemics of obesity and chronic illness move into neighborhoods across America. Instead of celebrating and modeling the lifestyle habits of women like Lori, we loathe them, and wish they'd move their skinny energetic butts somewhere else so we didn't have to look at them. This wish may soon be a reality as women across the country trade in their fruit salads for potato chips and their home gyms for home theaters.

Chapter 5

Healthy Meals for Busy Women

Rarely does a day go by that a woman doesn't stop to ask me what I eat. When I reply with, "I eat whatever I want; you know, real foods like quiche, chili, casseroles, tacos, steak, lasagna, soups, cookies, waffles, salads, fruit, and cobblers." Such a response is generally met with looks of disbelief. Twenty years ago, such looks surprised me; today however, I expect nothing less.

American women have been effectively marketed by processed food manufacturers and the diet industry to think that *real foods* are the reason they are sick, fatigued, and overweight. As we learned in Chapter 2, lies become truth as women listen to such propaganda and get lost in the toxic cloud of dietary confusion created by these industries.

Therefore, as you read the menus on the following pages do not be surprised by the absence of such items as rice cakes, fat-free salad dressing, low-fat cookies, or meal replacement shakes and bars, or low-carb potato chips, because I do not eat these lifeless foods, nor do I recommend them. What you will find are delicious, healthy meals prepared from fresh whole-food ingredients; meals that do not take long to prepare and pack well for snacks and lunches on the go.

Sample Breakfast Meals

(* recipe included)

- Omelet filled with raw cheese, avocado, tomatoes, olives; grapefruit
- Oatmeal with raw butter, raw milk/cream, raisins and cinnamon, 100% maple syrup; scrambled eggs
- Homemade granola* topped with raw milk and butter
- Leftover tri-tip (steak), potatoes, sliced tomatoes and red peppers, olives; sprouted bread
- Pork chop, leftover whole-grain cornbread, celery and peanut butter.
- Scrambled eggs, bowl of mixed fresh fruit, organic nitrate-free bacon, sprouted manna bread
- Leftover tomato soup, homemade whole-grain muffin
- Seasonal breakfast cobbler,* scrambled eggs, nitrate-free bacon or sausage.
- Waffles with butter and organic raw maple syrup, or topped with your favorite fruit; scrambled eggs
- Breakfast quiche,* sliced fresh tomatoes, fresh fruit of choice.
- Baked yam or sweet potato topped with butter and cinnamon, nitrate-free bacon or sausage, sliced raw vegetables
- Power Muffins* with raw cream
- French Toast made from sprouted bread topped with pure maple syrup

Sample Lunch Meals

- Grilled cheddar cheese and tomato sandwich; spinach salad with almonds
- Potato/Leek soup, sprouted sourdough bread and butter, coleslaw
- Sliced turkey, corn on the cob, apple, mixed salad and dressing
- Steak, pinto beans, broccoli/red pepper salad, corn tortillas
- Chicken tacos topped with cheese, lettuce, tomatoes, avocado; pinto beans
- Split pea soup,* pear, olives, sliced fresh vegetables, sprouted sourdough bread
- Tuna sandwich made with organic expeller-pressed mayonnaise, eggs, onions, celery; raw mixed-color vegetables, grapes
- Tostados filled with your favorite left-over meat, topped with mixed salad greens, large chunks of red peppers, olives, pinto beans, raw cheddar, guacamole
- Tomato & basil* with asparagus soup, tuna sandwich

Sample Dinner Meals

- Scallops, baked potatoes, mixed salad, glass of red wine
- Chili beans with cornbread
- Grilled chicken and pineapple, baked sweet potatoes, salad and dressing.
- Acorn squash/broccoli soup,* organic pork chop, sliced raw veggies, whole-grain bread
- Pot roast, baked potatoes, grilled zucchini, mixed salad
- Grilled salmon and red peppers, coleslaw, brown rice
- Spinach quiche,* tomato soup, mixed salad
- Grilled salmon, baked potatoes, Greek salad
- Meat loaf* with whipped potatoes and mixed salad
- Chicken kebabs, acorn squash, mixed salad, sour dough bread
- Grilled steak, coleslaw,* pinto beans, salsa

Cristi's Favorite Desserts

- Berry cobbler*
- Coconut Orange cookies*
- Carrot Cake
- Freshly made popcorn (cooked on the stove in coconut oil then topped with raw butter and a dash of sea salt).
- Cheesecake made with fresh raw crème cheese (fabulous)
- Peanut Butter Cookies

When Things Get Hectic

If I know that I am going to be extremely busy during a particular week I prepare my family's food ahead of time. This helps insure that we have plenty of food "ready to eat" during the week. When deciding on the menu, I like to choose things that can be easily converted into boxed-meals on the run: such as roast, stews, chili beans, deviled eggs, oatmeal cookies, chicken legs, mixed raw vegetables, fruit cobblers, and celery and peanut butter. I also prepare whole-grain muffins on Sunday evenings in addition to stirring up a large batch of homemade waffle mix for quick and delicious breakfasts.

Ladies, I encourage you to adopt a system of preparing your family's weekly meals ahead of time. We prepare food as described above on a regular basis; it is a habit that is built into our lives. The value in preparing meals in this fashion becomes quite evident come Monday morning, when you wake up to a refrigerator full of delicious and nutritious foods that will take carry you through most of the week without additional cooking.

The take home:

- Plan ahead
- Prepare ahead
- Share meal preparation with neighbors, friends, and family.
- You may have to drive out to a nearby farm for the healthiest food. It is worth it! Pack a lunch, load up the family, throw an ice-chest in the trunk, and make the gathering of nutritious foods a family event.

- When you do cook, make sure you prepare enough food to cover several meals over the next few days. Think large pots of chili and soups, whole chickens, large casseroles, grilled meats, quiche, etc.
- Double your cookie recipes and freeze half of the dough for use later.
- Wash all fresh fruits and vegetables, then slice and store in airtight containers ready for sack lunches or snacking.

With some basic ingredients kept on hand at all times, you will be able to create healthy meals your family will love;. Foods, whose innate flavors, colors, textures, and aromas, offer a sensory experience unmatched by processed foods that can go with you to work, school, the soccer field, or anywhere your busy lives may take you.

Some of Cristi's Favorite Recipes

The following original recipes are from my own kitchen. These recipes are simple to prepare, tasty, and nutritious. The amount listed for each ingredient is just an approximation, as I do not measure anything when I cook; I simply cannot cook that way. With that said, I have made each of these recipes countless times; thus, the measurements listed are pretty darn close. Besides, variation keeps things interesting and will allow you to add your own creativity.

*I have enlarged the font size for ease in reading during preparation

Quiche

1½ cups raw cream or milk
5 eggs
2 tablespoons melted raw butter
Juice from one lemon
1 ½ cups grated raw cheese (cheddar, Swiss, etc)
½- ¾ cup whole grain baking mix or whole grain flour
plus some baking powder
Cinnamon

Extras: Try adding raisins, frozen fresh berries, or
fresh spinach, nitrate-free sausage or bacon

Beat everything together in a large bowl. Pour into *a*
buttered baking dish and bake at 350° until set and
edges are brown. If you have a large family you will
want to double or triple this recipe so that there are
plenty of leftovers.

Creamy Pineapple Dressing
Over Sliced Cucumbers and Red Onions

1 cup whole plain organic yogurt or Kefir
1 ½ -2 cups chopped fresh pineapple
1 teaspoon coriander
½ teaspoon ground cloves
½ teaspoon chopped fresh ginger
½ cup olive oil
1/3 Balsamic vinegar

Puree in blender. Let chill for about 30 minutes.

Granola

Whenever I make granola it always turns out different. That's what makes it fun to prepare and a treat to eat. Most of the ingredients used are staples in my kitchen so that I can whip it up as needed. I eat these granola variations with raw milk or cream for breakfast, atop homemade ice cream, and sprinkled over baked apples. I take it along with me during all of my extended outdoor exercise excursions, and snack on it between meals or during weight training sessions. My three dogs also enjoy this healthy snack after long runs or during extended hiking trips. I encourage you to use your imagination and have fun making your own signature granola.

Basic ingredients:

1 cup unsalted melted butter
The juice from one lemon
1 jar organic raw nut butter (cashew, almond etc)
Approx. 1 cup or so of either milk, or yogurt
Approx. 2 cups of any organic whole-grain baking mix
Remember, variety is what keeps this recipe fun.

At this point, you can add such things as:

Seasonal or frozen berries
bananas, apples
chopped nuts
raisins, dates, other dried fruits
raw honey
nutmeg, cinnamon, allspice, etc.

Mix all ingredients together in a large bowl. Then, either form into 2 inch balls and place on a cookie sheet or, spread the entire mixture across a cookie sheet.

Bake in a 300° oven until lightly browned on top. When the granola is cool, remove from cookie sheet with a spatula breaking it up into pieces; store in an air-tight container or zip-lock bag.

Granola Recipe #2

1 stick butter
1 cup almond butter
1 cup apple juice
½ cup raw honey
1 tsp. cinnamon
2 cups oats
1 cup plain yogurt
2 chopped apples
1 cup flour
1 cup shredded raw coconut
2 eggs

Mix all ingredients together in a large bowl. Spread the Bake in a 300° oven until lightly browned on top. When the granola is cool, remove from cookie sheet with a spatula breaking it up into pieces; store in an air-tight container or zip-lock bag.

Potato Leek Soup

In medium cooking pot combine:

1 carton Pacific organic free-range chicken broth
5-6 chopped unpeeled potatoes
1 large chopped leek
Spices as desired

Cook until potatoes are soft.

Split Pea Soup

In medium cooking pot combine:

1 carton Pacific free-range low-salt chicken broth
1 cup water
1 bag dried peas
Spices as desired

Simmer on low heat for about forty-five minutes or until peas are soft. Mash and serve as is or with crumbled nitrate-free bacon.

.

Tomato & Basil with Asparagus Soup

1 pound of ground free-range turkey (cooked)
¾ carton of Pacific chicken broth
1 bunch of washed asparagus
1 large jar Walnut Acres Organic Tomato & Basil
Pasta Sauce.

In blender puree the broth and asparagus. Next, combine cooked turkey, broth mixture, and pasta sauce in a large cooking pot. Stir and simmer for about 15 minutes.

Seasonal Breakfast Cobbler

Chop up a large bowl about 2 cups of your favorite seasonal fruits:

In a separate large bowl combine
1 cup flax meal
1 cup oats
1 cup whole-grain baking mix
Allspice

Stir in:
1 cup melted butter
Juice from one fresh lemon
1 cup chopped nuts
1 cup or so of raw milk
Pour into a buttered baking dish and bake at 350° until browned.

Power Muffins

Muffins, like granola, offer a great opportunity for you to use whatever whole food ingredients are in your kitchen along with your imagination.

In a large mixing bowl combine two cups of any combination of whole grain flours or baking mix. If you are not using baking mix add one tablespoon of baking powder.

Stir in ½ cup Sucanat
spices (cinnamon or whatever you prefer)
2 eggs
Juice from one lemon
½ cup melted organic raw butter
1 cup or so of organic raw milk

Now add whatever is on hand:

Chopped pecans, walnuts, almonds, grated carrots, crushed pineapple, chopped apples, raisins, dates, figs, orange peel, blueberries, blackberries

Pour into buttered muffin tins and bake. Like the granola, these are great to take with you when you leave the house.

Acorn Squash and Broccoli Soup

In medium cooking pot combine:

1 carton Pacific Acorn Squash Soup
3 cups chopped Broccoli
1 teaspoon nutmeg
1 tablespoon grated orange peel

Simmer until Broccoli in tender. Serve alone or add grilled chicken.

Meatloaf

Combine in a large bowl:

2 or more pounds of ground organic free-range or grass-fed turkey, beef, or buffalo
1 ½ cups oats
1 or more cups chopped onion/ bell peppers etc
¼ cup organic brown mustard
2 eggs
1teaspoon garlic powder
1 teaspoon dried oregano
1 teaspoon dried basil
1 jar organic low-salt tomato sauce or Seeds of Change salsa

Bake at 350° for about an hour.

Coleslaw

Combine in large bowl:

4 or more cups shredded purple and green cabbage
4-6 shredded carrots
1 cup raisins (sulfur- free)
the juice from 2 lemons
cinnamon and coriander
½ cup Balsamic vinegar
1 cup or so Spectrum Naturals mayonnaise

Mix and chill over night

Stove Popped Popcorn

Popcorn
Organic coconut oil (this makes fantastic popcorn)
Sea salt

Gazpacho

1 carton Pacific chicken broth
10-15 fresh tomatoes
3-5 large multi-color bell peppers
2 cloves or more garlic
1 onion
1 peach
1 ½ cups cubed cantaloupe
1 can no-salt Muir Glenn tomato paste
1 tablespoon dried oregano

Gazpacho continued...

3 slices toasted sourdough bread
½ cup olive oil
2 tablespoons Balsamic vinegar
Juice from one lemon

Pour in batches into blender and blend on low. Continue until all ingredients have been combined. Serve with raw cream if desired.

Baked Salmon

Rinse salmon filet and place in a baking dish. Spread melted butter over the top of the filet and sprinkle moderately with whole-grain flour or baking mix. Next, sprinkle moderately with garlic powder, paprika, and oregano. Finally, drizzle the top with 2 tablespoons Balsamic Vinegar and the juice from 1 lemon. Bake at 325° until brown (about an hour).

Serve with whipped yams topped with cinnamon and crushed pineapple, a mixed salad, and a glass of your favorite wine if desired.

Summer Lentil Soup (delicious)

Step 1
Bring to boil 1 carton Pacific chicken broth, 1 cup water, and 1 16 oz. bag of red lentils. Reduce heat and simmer until tender about 1 hour.

Step 2
To blender add approximately half of the cooked lentils plus 1/3 cup olive oil, plus 4-5 fresh tomatoes, 2-3 bell peppers, and 1-2 cloves of garlic. Repeat step 2 with remaining lentils.

Once all of your blended ingredients have been combined into one bowl, stir in about 2 tablespoons Balsamic vinegar, the juice from one lemon, and sprinkle with paprika. Stir. Serve warm.

Flax Meal Crackers

Combine in large bowl:
2-cups flax meal
1 cup whole wheat flour
1/2 cup olive oil
1 tablespoon garlic powder
1 teaspoon cayenne powder
Hot water

Stir until it has the consistency of pie crust dough.

With floured hands separate into balls approximately the size of your fist. With a rolling pin, flatten each ball on floured wax paper and place on a cooking sheet greased with olive oil. Brush tops with butter and sprinkle with sea salt. Bake at 350° until brown and crispy on the ends.

Serve with hummus or your favorite spread.

Rosemary and Italian Parsley Dressing

½ cup olive oil
1 cup whole plain organic yogurt or kefir
Juice from 2 lemons
1tablespoon ground rosemary
1 bunch Italian parsley
1 banana
½ cup water

Puree all ingredients in blender. Serve the same day. My family loves this dressing over a bed of Spring mixed greens and topped with sliced red bell peppers.

Creamy Balsamic Vinaigrette

2 cups whole plain organic yogurt or kefir
1/4 cup balsamic vinegar
2 teaspoons black pepper
1 teaspoon coriander
Juice and zest from on lemon
1 cup olive oil
2 tablespoon ground basil

Puree all ingredients in blender. Chill for at least an hour before serving. Dressing will keep three to four days in a sealed container. Shake before serving. My family loves this dressing served over Greek salad.

Avocado Dressing and Sauce

2 cups spinach
Juice and zest from 2 lemons
1 cup olive oil
1 tablespoon chili powder
2 tablespoons apple cider vinegar
1 teaspoon peeled fresh garlic
1 teaspoon black pepper
1 teaspoon cayenne pepper
2 avocados
½ cup water if needed to puree

Puree all ingredients in blender. Chill for at least 30 minutes. We serve this sauce with tacos and other Mexican favorites and any mixed salad.

Coconut and Orange Cookies

In a large mixing bowl, cream together:
1 cup softened butter
½ cup Rapadura
1 egg
1 teaspoon pure vanilla extract
½ cup sour crème or whole plain yogurt
2 tablespoon grated peel from and organic orange

Stir in:
1 cup coconut
1 ½ cups oats
1 cup whole wheat graham flour
1 cup finely chopped pecans

Coconut Orange Cookies continued...

Thoroughly stir all ingredients. Place heaping spoonfuls onto an un-greased baking sheet. Bake in a 325 degree oven until browned around the edges (about 8 minutes).

Variations: I also like to add chopped organic dried fruits along with another egg into the mixture and put all of the dough into an oblong non-stick baking pan. Smooth the dough with a spatula and bake for about 20 minutes. Cut into bars.

Yankee Pot Roast

Large grass-fed roast
1½ cups Pacific beef broth
1/3 cup 100% whole wheat flour
2 tablespoons olive oil
½ cup raisins
1 cup chopped onion
1 ½ teaspoons curry powder
1 tablespoon garlic powder
½ teaspoon pepper
1 teaspoon allspice

Cover roast in flour. In a skillet, brown roast on all sides in olive oil. Combine remaining ingredients and pour over roast. Cover and bake at 350° for 3 hours or until meat is tender.

Sausage Skillet

2 large organic Kielbasa sausages
(I use Wellshire Farms)
2 large potatoes, sliced
2 large onions, sliced

In a large skillet, brown the sausages in about 1 cup of water. After the sausages are browned, remove them from the pan, but do not discard the drippings. Immediately add the potatoes and the onions into the sausage drippings and cook until tender and lightly brown. Add small amounts of water as needed if the liquid cooks out before the potatoes are tender. Combine all of the cooked ingredients into one pan and simmer until ready to serve.

Black Bean Dip

1 bag dry black beans (soaked, cooked, mashed)
½ cup olive oil
½ cup green onions chopped
1 tablespoon ground cumin
2 tablespoon red chili powder
½ cayenne powder (add more if you like it hotter)
1 jar Seeds of Change Salsa
1 cup chopped cilantro
½ cup chopped olives

Blend together in a bowl and serve with warm tortillas, organic corn chips, with chopped vegetables, or aside your favorite Mexican dishes.

Fresh Tomato and Corn Salsa
A Summer Favorite

3 ears of fresh corn cut from the cob
6 large ripe tomatoes chopped
2 jalapeño peppers diced
1 large diced cucumber
1 chopped red onion
1 large diced red bell pepper
1/4 cup chopped cilantro
Juice from 1 fresh lime
½ teaspoon sea salt
3 cloves chopped garlic

Combine ingredients on an air tight bowl. Chill for about an hour before serving to let the flavors blend.

Red Pepper Soup

2 red bell peppers, quartered and seeded
1 large sweet onion, peeled, cut in 1/2" wedges
2 cloves garlic, peeled and halved
1/2 tsp. dried thyme
1 tsp. extra virgin olive oil
1 carton organic chicken broth
1 can Glenn Muir organic whole tomatoes
1 bag frozen organic corn kernels
freshly ground black pepper to taste
1/4 cup fresh cilantro leaves or chopped basil, optional

continued...

Bring all ingredients to a boil. Reduce heat immediately and simmer on low until vegetables are soft, but not mushy.

Fresh Mexican Soup

5 cups water
1 whole organic chicken
1 cup chopped carrots
1 cup chopped bell pepper
1 cup chopped onion
1 cup chopped zucchini
1 cup sliced celery
1 small can Muir Glenn organic tomato paste
2 teaspoons fresh or dried oregano
1 tablespoon fresh or ground cumin
1/2 cup brown uncooked rice

1 bunch fresh cilantro, chopped fine, divided in half
1 lb. grass-fed lean ground beef
1 egg
Sea salt and pepper to taste
Chopped green onions

Place washed whole chicken in the water in a large pot. Cover and boil until chicken falls easily off the bone. Pout broth through a strainer; reserve all of the broth.

Separate the bones from the chicken; discard bones. Return the chicken and the broth to the large cooking pot. Add the next ten ingredients and simmer on low.

Meanwhile, in a large bowl, mix ground beef, egg, remaining cilantro, along with the salt and pepper. Brown in a skillet until the meat is fully cooked. Drain any excess grease, and add the meat to the large cooking pot. Simmer until ready to serve.

Sprinkle green onion on top of soup before serving.

Coconut and Chicken Chowder

Olive oil for browning chicken
3 chicken breast halves, diced
2 large red peppers, seeded and diced
1 large green onion, thinly sliced
1 large clove garlic, minced
1 can organic coconut milk
1 box organic chicken broth
1/4 cup creamy natural peanut butter
2 teaspoons hot sauce
1 1/4 teaspoons sea salt

Brown diced chicken in olive oil until fully cooked and tender. Drain as needed.

In a large cooking pot combine all ingredients including the cooked chicken. Simmer on low for about 15 minutes.

Fruit Cobbler

Pre-heat oven to 350 degrees

Filling:
6-8 cups sliced apple, nectarines, or peaches
Juice from one lemon
½ cup chopped pecans
½ cup raisins
Cinnamon

Crust:
1 stick butter, melted
½ cup Sucanat
1 cup raw milk
½ cup oats
1 cup whole-grain baking mix
Cinnamon

Slice thoroughly washed unpeeled fruit and place in a 2 quart baking dish. Add the pecans and raisins, and stir. Pour the lemon juice over the fruit and sprinkle with cinnamon.

Prepare crust batter by mixing all ingredients together in a bowl. Pour over fruit and bake until golden brown on top.

Simply Delicious Spinach Spread

This spread is easy and delicious. Spread it liberally on your favorite whole grain bread or flax crackers!
1 bag pre-washed spinach leaves
2 cloves garlic, minced
1 onion, chopped
2 tablespoon cold-pressed olive oil
2 tablespoon flax oil
1 1/2 cups kefir (or sour cream)
Pinch nutmeg
Sea salt and freshly ground pepper to taste

Blanch the spinach in boiling water for two minutes. Sauté garlic, onion and well-drained spinach in the olive oil for three minutes on low heat. Put sautéed mixture and the rest of the ingredients into a blender and mix on pulse setting for a chunky spread.

Parsley Mayonnaise

Serve this versatile mayonnaise with a platter of raw vegetables such as carrot or celery sticks, sliced cucumber, radishes, broccoli and cauliflower florets, or as a sauce with cooked potatoes.

1/2 cup yogurt or kefir
Juice from 1 lemon
1 teaspoons mustard
1 tablespoon flax seed oil
1/2 teaspoon balsamic vinegar
1 teaspoon onion powder

1/4 clove garlic, minced
1/2 teaspoon sea salt
1 tablespoon parsley, finely chopped
1/4 cup cream cheese

Blend all ingredients in a blender until emulsified.

Lemon-Chive Vinaigrette
Over Middle Eastern Couscous Salad

For the vinaigrette:
Juice from 2 lemons
¼ cup olive oil
½ teaspoon sea salt
½ teaspoon freshly ground black pepper
1 teaspoon curry powder
1 teaspoon garlic powder
4 tablespoons chopped chives
2 tablespoons Balsamic vinegar

For the salad:
2 cups Middle Eastern Couscous, cooked and cooled
1 red onion, thinly sliced
1 large red pepper, sliced into thin strips
1 cup cherry tomatoes, halved
4 cucumber, peeled and diced
1 cup chopped scallions

Combine the salad ingredients.
Stir in vinaigrette and chill for about 30 minutes.

Pineapple-Ginger Chutney

1 ½ cups fresh pineapple, chopped
½ cup organic raisins
2 teaspoons fresh ginger, finely chopped
Juice and zest from 1 lime
1 teaspoon sea salt

Combine all ingredients in a jar with a tight lid. Store in refrigerator for 2-3 days; serve as a side dish with fish or chicken.

Black Bean, Fresh Corn
And Red Pepper Salad

1/3 cup cider vinegar
1 tablespoon coarse-grained mustard
2 tablespoons olive oil
1/2 sea salt
1/4 teaspoon freshly ground black pepper
1 small red onion, diced
1 bag black beans, soaked, cooked, and cooled
Corn from 2 fresh ears, cooked and cooled
1 large red bell pepper, trimmed and sliced
2 tablespoons fresh parsley, chopped

Combine all ingredients in an air tight bowl and chill for about and hour.

Fall Spinach Salad with Pears and Pecans

For the vinaigrette:
1 tablespoon finely chopped shallots
1 tablespoon organic Dijon mustard
1 tablespoon melted raw honey
3 tablespoons red wine vinegar
¼ cup olive oil
¼ cup apple cider vinegar

For the salad:
4-6 cups baby spinach leaves
2 sliced pears
1/2 cup dried natural cranberries
1 tablespoon chopped pecans

Combine all ingredients in a jar with a tightly secured lid.. Refrigerate for 24 hours before serving. Tangy!

Mobile Fitness Bars

Say goodbye to processed energy bars and hello to homemade goodness with this recipe for my favorite nutrition bars. I make these bars to take when we go on long outings where I know they are going to get tossed in the bottom of a daypack or jack pocket. My dogs love them also.

½ cup melted butter
½- ¾ cup plain yogurt
The juice and zest from 2 lemons

½ cup flax meal
1 ½ - 2 cups chopped dried date, prunes, or figs
(sulfur-free)
1 cup finely chopped walnuts or pecans
½ cup oats
1 cup whole-grain baking mix
or
1 cup Bob's Red Mill graham flour plus 2 teaspoons
baking powder

Mix first three ingredients together in a large bowl.
Stir in the dry ingredients, followed by the dries fruit
and nuts.

Pour into a buttered 8X8 non-stick pan, and bake at
350 degrees for 20-25 minutes.

This final recipe has been reprinted from the January
2006 issue of my monthly newsletter "Ideas for Healthy
Living". Go to www.cristidoll.com to join my family of
readers.

Ideas for Healthy Living
January 2006

By: Cristi J. Doll, Ph. D.

This issue is going to address the topic of
detoxification, or cellular cleansing. I know your first
reaction is to think to yourself: "What the heck is she going
to ask me to do?" Let me fire back by saying, I am NOT
going to ask you to do anything weird, or at least too weird.
But let's face it, there aren't too many of us who couldn't

stand a bit of internal housekeeping following the November through December feeding frenzy.

Why Detoxify?

- To increase energy and enhance health
- To help those desiring to lose weight (very important to success)
- To improve sleep
- To help "de-gunk" the intestines (and cells) following extended periods of poor eating.
- To enhance a woman's ability to conceive and have a healthy pregnancy
- To help our bodies remove potentially dangerous chemicals obtained from the environment

A Simple and Effective Way to Help the Body Eliminate Toxins...

Eat more vegetables!!!

It should come as no surprise that few among us consume enough fresh produce, particularly vegetables. With this in mind, I am going to introduce you to a convenient and tasty way to increase the number of fruits and vegetables you eat each day...in our house we call them Green Magma Vitality Drinks. These drinks are great ways to increase your vegetable intake and are one powerhouse of a smoothie* created by pureeing a variety of fresh fruits and vegetables in a blender.

And yes you read is correctly, I said blender, not juicer. I am not a proponent of juicers as they remove the natural fibers. In case you have been hiding under a rock for the past 50 years, colon cancer and other intestinal disorders (yes, constipation is a colon disorder) are wide spread. All of those wonderful soluble and insoluble fibers found in fresh fruits, vegetables, and whole grains act as brooms to go through and help clean the inside of the colon, and as softeners to help things move through more easily.

After consuming these Vitality Drinks for a few days, you will understand why I say they are one of my top picks for internal housekeeping. Most people report that once they get past the greenness of these drinks, they love them, and feel much better when such Daily Vitality Drinks are a regular part of their day. In fact, the universal response is, "Wow! I had no clue that something this simple could make me feel so good; I can really tell that the "junk" is leaving my body."

Question: "Will this smoothie taste like the ones I make with milk, chocolate syrup, and frozen fruit?"

Answer: When I put an asterisk beside the word smoothie above, I did so because the sample recipe that follows is by no stretch of the imagination going to taste like a milkshake. (In fact, I strongly suggest that you refrain from adding milk to these types of drinks).

Green Magma Daily Vitality Drink

Fill blender approximately half way with filtered water. Next, begin adding washed and peeled (when necessary) fresh fruits (or frozen) and fresh vegetables about a cup or so at a time, blending on high between each addition. I recommend using only one cup of fruit, and the remainder vegetables, as the intent is to make these primarily veggie, not fruit drinks. Too much fruit at one time can spike your blood-sugar and sabotage your weight loss (if this applies to you). Stop adding ingredients when the blender is full (duh). It doesn't really matter which fruits or vegetables you use, except that I would shy away from selecting anything with sharp pieces such as asparagus.

I like to use black berries, blue berries, strawberries, banana, apple, papaya, guava, and pineapple, preferably seasonal, and organic where available. Remember, limit fruit to approx. one cup, or one whole banana, apple, pear, etc.

My Vitality Drinks are largely spinach. For convenience, I use the pre-washed spinach in bags found in the cold box in the produce section of most grocery stores. The remaining vegetables I wash and cut into chunks or handfuls such as celery, beets, parsley, kale, tomatoes, broccoli, cauliflower, cabbage, and other greens. Rotate the vegetables and fruits you use so as to insure a wide variety of nutrients. I DO NOT recommend garlic or onions in this type of drink, as it doesn't do much for the taste and smell tends to linger in the blender.

Use your imagination, blend well, and enjoy a Daily Vitality Drink.

Cookbook Modifications

With any cookbook recipe I make the following modifications:

- Replace white flour with whole grain flours
- Use whole-grain pastas in moderation
- Be very careful when selecting sauces, broth, soups, and dressings, many are full of salt, sugars (high fructose corn syrup), and preservatives. It is much better to purchase these items from health food and specialty grocers that carry higher quality packaged foods and read the labels carefully.
- Buy dried beans instead of canned and soak overnight prior to slow cooking
- Eliminate refined sugars and drastically reduce ALL sweeteners.
- Always use fresh fruits and vegetables whenever available instead of canned or frozen.
- Do not use any artificial sweeteners
- Never use vegetable oils, margarine, or shortening in your cooking. Instead choose (salt-free butter, flax meal, olive oil, or coconut oil)
- Use salt-free seasonings or sea salt and fresh herbs
- Avoid all processed deli style meats except nitrate-free (the internet is a great source for this information).

Chapter 6

The Busy Woman's Guide to Weight Loss and Fitness

I wonder if our ancestors sat around the campfire counting calories or carbs, blowing up their stability balls, or analyzing the glycemic index? I wonder if they tried creating meal-replacement shakes or bars, or went in search of fat-free walnut trees or cows that gave low-fat milk?

Our world is quickly filling up with women (and men) struggling to lose weight. They are in fast pursuit of that miracle diet or program that will result in a smaller body and better health. Sadly, instead of adopting lifestyle habits that promote a healthy, lean, energetic body (whole foods, a progressive fitness program, adequate rest, fulfilling relationships, meaningful work) they run themselves ragged with overcommitted schedules that leave little time to procure nutritious foods, exercise regularly, rest their tired bodies, and nurture their spirits.

Ladies, middle-age spread is not something that just happens as a result of aging or a slow metabolism. All of those extra pounds are earned and your metabolism is made sluggish by years of poor food and lifestyle choices. The results are cumulative. Poor health and the extra ten, twenty-five, or fifty pounds do not suddenly happen because you ate a Twinkie yesterday and skipped your workout. Diabetes, heart disease, and middle-age spread for example, result from years of poor food choices and skipped workouts. Likewise, being healthy, lean, and energetic also the result from lifestyle habits that are cumulative. Vibrant health will not magically happen because you ate your broccoli yesterday and took a short walk.

Give your body the fuel it needs when it needs it.

Our bodies require a wide variety of nutrient dense foods in quantities necessary for growth and repair, and to support the workloads we place upon them. Excess food (fuel), even from high quality foods, will store as fat if we consume beyond what is necessary to keep our bodies functioning efficiently and to meet the physical demands placed upon them.

So how can we solve this problem without counting calories? Simple, give your body the fuel it needs when it needs it. Although your body needs a wide variety of whole nutrient dense foods to maintain good health, certain foods are not necessary in large quantities if you lead a sedentary lifestyle or during long periods of inactivity. These foods, specifically grains, starchy vegetables, desserts, and yes girls…too much fruit, can convert easily to body fat if not used up during activity.

Here is how I apply this principle to my own life:

During a typical week, my fuel requirements are high. I strength train four to five times each week, and participate in many of the following activities: walking or running my three dogs, mountain biking, sprint training, dancing, hiking, gardening, swimming, and roller skating. As a result, my body needs a constant supply of proteins, fats, and carbohydrates. I eat a combination of these micronutrients every time 2-4 hours (note sample menus in Chapter 5). I adjust the amount of food I eat throughout the day to meet the physical demands I place on my body. On days when I am not training and my physical demands are low, my meals are much smaller. Again, the foods themselves do not change, only the quantities.

Here are some examples. During mountain biking season my husband and I ride three days each week. Our rides are usually quite strenuous, lasting anywhere from one to two hours, as we climb 10-15 miles up and down rocky terrain. If we ride in the mornings, I will usually eat a large stack of whole-grain pancakes topped with butter and real maple syrup, 3-4 pieces of nitrate-free organic bacon or a pork chop, a glass of raw milk, and a piece of fruit. During the ride if I get hungry I snack on fruit and nuts, or one of my homemade power bars. If we are going to ride after dinner, I will eat a serving of meat, a baked potato with butter, a salad, 2 pieces of sourdough bread, and one of my homemade desserts. Again, this is prior to strenuous exercise be it mountain biking, weight training, or other activities requiring a sufficient amount of fuel.

On non-training days or days of light activity we eat smaller meals and usually drop all manmade carbohydrates such as breads, and desserts. Even though we only eat healthy nutritious breads and desserts, our bodies do not need this type of fuel. In the absence of strenuous activity such foods are easily converted into body fat. Thus, a typical non-workout breakfast might include a scrambled egg, 1-2 pieces of nitrate-free organic bacon, and a half of grapefruit. Later for lunch, we might have some leftover chicken, a small serving of homemade potato salad, and some raw vegetables. You will notice that there are no grains, desserts, and only small amounts of starch. We do not eat meal replacement bars or any other processed foods to meet our day fuel needs. We simply adjust the amount of food we eat to the amount of activity we are going to get, and take extra food with us on all of our outings.

Now, how might this work in your life? Let's say that tomorrow you are scheduled to get up early and head to the gym to lift weights and do some sprint training. For breakfast, you might have a couple of pieces of French toast made with sprouted whole-grain bread and organic eggs topped with raw butter and pure maple syrup, 2-3 pieces of nitrate-free organic bacon or sausage, and maybe a piece of fruit. Following your workout you should have a snack that contains nutrients for replenishment and muscle growth; I would suggest a piece of fresh fruit, a slice of raw cheese, and a handful of almonds. If you were not planning to exercise in the morning, you might opt for an omelet filled with raw cheese and chopped vegetables, and a half of grapefruit. Since you are not training, there is no need for bread or heavy starches.

Now, let's say that you sit behind a desk all day for work. When you pack your lunches and snacks the night before, you will want to chose a protein, such as chicken, fish, or beef, tuna; some healthy fat such as a handful of olives or raw nuts, a few pieces of raw cheese, a large salad containing a variety of raw vegetables, and a couple of pieces of fruit. Since you will be sitting for an extended period of time, your body does not require the extra food energy from grains, desserts, or large amounts of starchy vegetables. Simply graze on the foods you bring with you during your breaks and at lunch in order to keep your blood-sugar balanced.

Next, let's say that three nights each week you attend a ninety-minute kick boxing class. During the day, your meals will be similar to the ones I just listed, but for dinner, you will want to add some starches such as potatoes, yams, or beans, and maybe some bread and dessert. Since you will be participating in strenuous physical activity, this is the time for those extra carbohydrates before your workout and as a post workout snack.

If on the remaining two week-nights you take a class after work and will be sitting for several hours, your dinner on these nights will want to resemble your lunches: a protein (chicken), some fat (raw cream sauce served over your chicken), mixed salad, along with a piece of fresh fruit. During your breaks you can snack on some raw nuts and raisins, or some almond butter and celery sticks.

Once this way of eating becomes a habit, it is really quite simple. I encourage you to plan your meals ahead of time, and adjust the quantity of food you eat to match your body's fuel needs throughout the day.

The Road to Success

1. Stop eating processed foods; these foods can damage your health, drain your energy, and interfere with the body's ability to lose weight.

2. Eat real whole-foods consumed as close to their natural state as possible. Such foods are full of vital nutrients that support vibrant health, increase energy, and help you to achieve a healthy weight without dieting.

3. Keep blood sugar balanced by not skipping meals. An efficient metabolism requires balanced blood-sugar. You can accomplish this by eating every three hours or so throughout the day and include plenty of healthy fats (nuts, olives, avocado etc). Fat signals your brain that it is satisfied; otherwise, you will crave carbohydrates and always be hungry.

4. Fitness conscious people understand the importance of meal frequency.

- Faster metabolic rate
- Higher energy levels
- Less storage of body fat due to smaller portions
- Reduced hunger and cravings

- Steadier blood sugar and insulin levels
- More calories usable for muscle growth

5. If you are going to be gone from the house for more than two hours...PACK A LUNCH. Do not give yourself a reason (or excuse) to skip meals or stop for junk food.

6. Prepare most of your food ahead of time so that you always have healthy food to take with you. Rarely do I leave my house without water and food.

7. Save your desserts and grains for just before and just after high intensity workouts or other periods of moderate or greater physical activity. This way, the simple sugars are used up by the body during and after exercise instead of being stored as fat.

8. If you consume any of The 10 Foods That Should Never Touch a Woman's Lips, you volunteer for your own weight challenges and strain your immune system which can lead to a host of health problems.

9. Do not count calories, carbohydrates, or fat grams. This is a complete waste of your valuable time and takes the pleasure out of eating.

10. Follow the sample menus in this book, and make adjustments to match your activity throughout the day.

Let's Get in Shape

The human body is designed to be used daily. Through movement we flex our muscles, massage lymph nodes, move the walls of blood vessels, provide stress to bones, and increase our heart rate. As a result, our bodies become stronger, more resilient, and better able to handle everyday movements like walking, sitting, and standing. Increasing the frequency and intensity of our movement allows our bodies to perform more challenging tasks: hiking, weight lifting, rollerblading, rock climbing, mountain biking, dancing, karate, gymnastics, water skiing, snow shoeing, and any other activities. For those who begin these activities in childhood and continue with them regularly as they age, life is pleasurable as they enjoy the fruits of their labor (a fit healthy body) well into their senior years.

Unfortunately, many women rarely participate in physical activity beyond daily tasks. When they do decide to begin exercising, they quickly discover that the programs they select do not result in the lean, fit body they desire. Thus, many conclude that exercise simply does not work for them.

As I stated above, exercise always works; however, as the body adapts to the new stimuli (workload) being placed upon it, the workload must change. Most women fail to grasp this point. Ladies, strolling down the block for twenty minutes three times per week is not going to cut it. When women complain to me that their fitness programs are not working, upon review I quickly ascertain that their activities are clearly low in intensity, short in duration, infrequent, and lack variety in order to challenge different muscle groups and energy systems. Therefore, if you want to continue getting results from your current fitness routine you need to mix things up from time to time. If walking is your preferred exercise, walk faster, walk farther, walk up hills, or better yet, add some different forms of exercise to your week such as: swimming, bike riding, yoga, martial arts, roller skating, or dancing.

Taking It to the Next Level of Fitness

After you have been exercising consistently as described above for three to six months, you are ready to take your fitness to the next level with the inclusion of anaerobic cardiovascular exercise along with a progressive strength training program.

Unfortunately, many women have never trained with weights and other forms of anaerobic exercise, or they haven't explored these fitness modalities enough to experience their benefits. Ladies, a well planned strength and anaerobic cardiovascular training program can enhance your health, increase your energy, and is critical in helping you achieving the lean, firm body you desire. Furthermore, it is your base (core) program that gets you in shape and keeps you in shape year round so that you can go hiking, dancing, skiing, mountain biking, roller skating, or any other physical activities you might like to participate in.

The weekly gym-based program I recommend to all of my clients who do not train with me one on one, is Phil Campbell's Ready, Set, Go! Synergy Fitness for Time Crunched Adults. After 20 years in this industry I have reviewed many different training programs and the Ready, Set, Go Program is by far one of the best. The instruction in this book is first rate. If you are looking for results, these workouts deliver. You will become your own personal trainer as you learn step by step how to synergize your metabolism, cut body fat, and tone and build muscle. Additionally, this program grows with you as you continually increase your fitness level. It is designed for beginners to advanced athletes, with a specific focus on the fitness challenges facing people during mid-life. After six months on this program, you will not recognize yourself. For more information, visit Phil's website at www.readysetgofitness.com.

No Gym, No Problem

When was the last time you...?

- Rode your bike
- Went to family night at your local skating rink
- Took a long walk at a local park
- Hiked in the mountains
- Went swimming
- Ran the track (or the stadium steps) at the local high school
- Ran sprints
- Did pushups or pull-ups
- Stretched
- Walked your dog
- Went dancing
- Took a yoga class
- Learned a form of martial arts
- Threw a ball with your kids
- Jumped rope

A Quick Note to Soccer Moms

When I use the term "Soccer Mom," I am referring to all mothers who sit on the sidelines watching their children's sports practices. Moms, this is the perfect opportunity for you and the other mothers to get *your* exercise.

When my now 22 year old son was growing up and playing sports I would walk, jog, jump rope, and run sprints somewhere around the perimeter of where his team was practicing. This allowed me to watch him and get in my own workout at the same time. On game days I sat with the other parents. He and I also participated in a variety of activities together over the years that we still engage in today both together and individually such as: mountain biking, rollerblading, family nights at the local roller skating rink, backpacking, martial arts, and country dancing.

Moms, when you exercise around and with your children, you not only enhance your own health, you help create lasting memories while instilling healthy habits in them that will likely carry over into adulthood.

Letters from Readers

The following letters were sent to me from two women after they (and their husbands) read The 10 Foods That Should Never Touch a Woman's Lips before this revised edition was released.

Be Powerful!
By: Casey S. Colsher

After 28 years, I have found it! What is it? Well, I have found the perfect balance in my life mentally and physically; I am at peace with who I am as a person. I was not always here, but I know that a good diet, regular exercise, and for me personally YOGA has been a huge contributor in my success.

It's true. As a new mom, with a nearly one year old daughter; I realize how important nutrition is in our lives. I vowed that I would feed my daughter right. I did not want her growing up eating fruits and vegetables sprayed with pesticides or meat and milk filled with hormones. Her little body is a temple and would be treated as such.

We made the move as a family to eat organically. It is one of the better decisions I have ever made. There is something to be said about eating naturally. I feel more satisfied and energetic than ever before. We can't wait to go to the grocery store and stock up on real, whole food. We eat healthy, colorful, fun meals, which in turn makes us feel healthy, colorful and fun!!!

I can't stress enough how much better I feel. I know that eating right is only one component and the other is exercise. Again, as an example to my daughter, my husband and I incorporate exercise into our daily lives. I can't wait to strap my daughter into her jogging stroller and go. If we are short on time, we walk around our neighborhood; if we have the day, we make a fun trip to a local park to enjoy the scenery and hit the tougher terrain.

I know our lives get crazy and bogged down, but the importance of making time to be active and eat right has to become a part of that. You will thank yourself for treating your body with respect. Why not do everything you can to better yourself and set an example for the people around you. Be powerful!!!

Cherish Your Body
By: Kristin Amrhein

Dear Dr. Doll,

I have always thought of myself as a healthy woman or should I say always concerned about my body's appearance. Now, at the age of 28 and a mother of two, I would say I still am concerned with my appearance, but on a completely different level. I have always wanted to be thin, or should I say thinner, no matter what expense I put my body through. This was especially true during high school and college. Skipping meals, diet pills, fad diets, inconsistent exercise patterns, etc. Now, over ten years later and after the life changing experience of having children, I finally get it.

It's not about being thin but appreciating your body. I now have learned to cherish my body. Instead of always yearning to be thinner, I yearn to be healthy. There is a major difference and as much as I wish I would have known this fact then I'm glad I do now. With this new understanding, I choose to show my body appreciation by treating it kindly with the right foods and proper exercise. My family and I eat organic meats, vegetables and fruits, and whole grains. We eat healthy snacks and well balanced meals. It makes me feel good to eat this way but mostly, it makes me feel better knowing that my children are also eating high quality food. I only hope that I can teach them early on to respect their bodies.

Exercise is a staple in our household. Life is hectic...period. I know this; everyone knows this. Each of us has a laundry list of things that need to get done in a day. I chose to place exercise at the top of that list. My children (ages 1 and 2) have grown to love the double jogging stroller. They know that if they are good while mommy gets her jog/walk in then they get rewarded with healthy snacks and time to run around at a park. If it's a rainy day or winter, I try to fit in my workouts during their nap time or after they go to bed. Sometimes my exercise sessions are long, sometimes they are short; either way, I believe that exercise makes me a better person, wife, and mom.

I am thankful that I FINALLY get it. I get the importance of real foods, exercising, and instilling these values into my family life. I am not perfect... believe me, and I still have a lot more to learn. One thing I know for sure, I want my family and I to be healthy and happy.

I'd like to thank you, Dr. Doll, for bringing awareness to me through your book, The 10 Foods. Since reading it, I have a better understanding of nutrition, and have changed many things. For example, I have given up diet sodas, artificial sweeteners such as Splenda, and have made the switch to mostly organic meats, fruits, and vegetables. With this new knowledge I feel empowered; but mostly I feel healthy!

Sincerely,

Kristin Amrhein

Parting Thoughts

Nutrient dense foods as nature intended them, together with lifestyle habits that support rejuvenation, contain miraculous restorative powers. Be mindful in selecting the highest quality foods for you and your family, as nutritious food lovingly prepared and consumed in a peaceful setting, is capable of nurturing our whole being. Revel in its magic!

We invite you to visit us at

www.cristidoll.com

for more great Ideas for Healthy Living!

Recommended Reading, Viewing, and Surfing

Reading

Fast Food Nation
By: Eric Schlosser (Perennial Publishers)

The Omnivore's Dilemma
By: Michael Pollan (Penguin Press)

Food Politics: How the Food Industry Influences Nutrition and Health
By: Marion Nestle (University of California Press)

The Untold Story of Milk
By: Ronald Schmid (New Trends Publishing)

Nutrition and Physical Degeneration.
By: Weston Price (Price-Pottenger Nutrition Foundation)

Excitotoxins: The Taste That Kills
By: Russell Blaylock (Health Press)

Nourishing Traditions.
By: Sally Fallon (New Trends Publishing)

Ready, Set, Go! Synergy Fitness for Time-Crunched Adults
By: Phil Campbell, MS, MA, FASHE (Pristine Publishers)

Viewing

Oscar Nominated *Super Size Me*
Written by: Morgan Spurlock

Surfing

www.westonaprice.org

www.organicpastures.com

www.eatwild.com

www.grasslandbeef.com

www.eatwellguide.org

www.readysetgofitness.com

www.realmilk.com

www.cafarmersmarkets.com

www.organicconsumers.org

www.ams.usda.gov/farmersmarkets/map.htm

www.biodynamics.com/csa.html

Sources Consulted

Allan, Christian B., and Wolfgang Lutz. Life Without Bread.
Los Angeles: Keats Publishing, 2000.

Baker, Sydney. Detoxification and Healing: The Key to
Optimal Health. New Canaan: Keats Publishing,
1997.

Ballentine, Rudolph. Diet & Nutrition. Honesdale: The
Himalayan International Institute, 1978.

Blaylock, Russell. Excitotoxins: The Taste That Kills. Santa
Fe New Mexico: Health Press, c1994.

Beyond Vegetarianism Contrary Facts Verses Vegan Dogma.
27 Dec. 2001.
http://www.beyonveg.com

Browen, Jim. "Splenda - Anything But Splendid." Rense.com. 20
Apr 2004 http://www.rense.com/general48/sps.htm.

Campbell, Phil. Ready, Set, Go! Synergy Fitness for Time-
Crunched Adults. Pristine Publishers, 2003.

Cassel, Ingri . "Splenda is not Splendid ." Nov 2003. Idaho
Observer. 20 Apr 2004.
http://proliberty.com/observer/20031112.htm

Census Bureau, Statistical Abstract of the United States. Section
3 Health and Nutrition. 2004-2005.
http://www.census.gov/prod/2002pubs/01statab/health.pdf.

Challem, Jack. Fructose, Maybe Not So Natural...Maybe Not So
Safe. The Nutritional Reporter, 1995.
http://www.nutrtionreporter.com

Critser, Greg. Fat Land: How Americans Became the Fattest People in the World . Boston: Houghton Mifflin Company, 2003.

Connelly, Scott A. Dr. Scott Connelly's 6-Pack Prescription. New York: The Berkley Publishing Group, 2001.

Crook, William G. The Yeast Connection Handbook. 1996. Jackson: Professional Books, 2002.

"Diet, Consumption, and Health." United States Department of Agriculture Economic Research Service web site, Oct 2004. http://www.ers.usda.gov/Topics/View.asp?T=101400.

Fallon, Sally. Nourishing Traditions. 1999. Washington: New Trends Publishing Inc., 2001.

Forristal, Linda Joyce, CCP, MTA. "In the Kitchen of Mother Linda: The Rise and Fall of Crisco." From the Weston A. Price Foundation website Dec. 2003. http://www.westonaprice.org/motherlinda/fats_crisco.html.

Francis, Raymond. Never Be Sick Again. Deerfield Beach: Health Communications, Inc., 2002.

Frost, Mary. Going Back to the Basics. 2nd ed. Mary Frost, 1997.

Gittleman, Ann Louise. Super Nutrition for Women. New York: Bantam Books, 1991.

Gittleman, Ann Louise. Get the Salt Out: 501 Simple Ways to Cut the Salt Out of Any Diet. New York: Three Rivers Press, 1996.

Gittleman, Ann Louise. Get the Sugar Out: 501 Simple Ways to Cut the Sugar Out of Any Diet. New York: Three Rivers Press, 1996.

Gold, Mark D. "The Bitter Truth About Artificial Sweeteners." Nexus Magazine, Volume 2, #28 (Oct-Nov 1995) and Volume 3, #1 (Dec 1995-Jan 1996). http://www.nexusmagazine.com/articles/aspartame.html.

Ifland, Joan. Sugars and Flours: How They Make Us Crazy, Sick and Fat, And What to do About It. 1st Books Library™, 2003.

Jensen, Bernard. Food Healing for Man. Escondido: Bernard Jensen International, 1983.

Jensen, Bernard. The Chemistry of Man. Escondido: Bernard Jensen International, 1983.

Jensen, Bernard. A New Lifestyle for Health & Happiness. Escondido: Bernard Jensen International, 1980.

Lipski, Elizabeth. Digestive Wellness. 1996. Los Angeles: Keats Publishing, 2000.

"Low Calorie Sweeteners : Sucralose." 2004. Calorie Control Council . 08 Apr 2004. http://www.caloriecontrol.org/sucralos.html.

Lydon, Christine. "Could There Be Evil Lurking in Aspartame Consumption?" Oxygen Magazine, Oct. 1999.

Martin, Jeanne Marie. Complete Candida Yeast Guidebook. Revised 2nd ed. Roseville: Prima Health, 2000.

McDonald's Quality & Nutrition Information McDonald's Corporation. 2004-2005. http://www.mcdonalds.com/usa/eat/nutrition_info.html

Mercola, Joseph. "The Potential Dangers of Sucralose." 2004.
Dr. Joseph Mercola. 08 Apr 2004.
http://www.mercola.com/2000/dec/3/sucralose_dangers.
htm.

Murray, Michelle W. "Salt: The Forgotten Killer." The
University of Maryland Web Site. 2005.
http://www.umm.ede/cgi-bin

Nestle, Marion. Food Politics: How the Food Industry Influences
Nutrition and Health. Berkley California: University of
California Press, 2002.

Payne, Cynthia. "Trans Fats 101." University of Maryland
Medical Center. 2004.
http://www.umm.edu/features/transfats/html.

Pick OB/GYN NP, Marcella. "Splenda-is it unsafe? Or truly the
perfect artificial sweetener?" Women to Women web
site 1998 - 2005.
http://www.womentowomen.com/LIBsplenda.asp.

Price, Weston. Nutrition and Physical Degeneration. 1939. La
Mesa: Price-Pottenger Nutrition Foundation, 2000.

Sanda, Bill. The Dangers of High Fructose Corn Syrup: from
Wise Traditions in Food, Farming, and the Healing Arts;
Winter 2003.
http://www.westonaprice.org/modernfood/fructose/http:

Schlosser, Eric. Fast Food Nation. New York: Perennial
Publishers, 2002.

Schmid, Ronald. Traditional Foods Are Your Best Medicine.
1987.   Rochester: Healing Art Press, 1997.

Simontacchi, Carol. The Crazy Makers: How the Food Industry
Is Destroying Our Brains and Harming Our Children.
New York: Penguin Putnam Inc. 2000.

Spencer, Fred MD. "Thermogenesis." Natural Health and Longevity Resource Center website. http://www.all-natural.com/thermo.html.

"Splenda Cooking and Baking Tips." 2002. Splenda: Low Carb Sweetener. McNeil UK. 21 Apr2004 www.splenda.co.uk.

Stoddard, Mary Nash. Deadly Deception - Story of Aspartame. Odenwald Press, 1998.

"Sucralose Toxicity Information Center." Holistic Medication. 08 Apr 2004. http://www.holisticmed.com/splenda/.

"Sucralose." 2004. International Sweeteners Association. 08 Apr 2004. http://www.isabru.org/frameset.html.

"The Only Low-Calorie Sweetener Made From Sugar." 8 April 2004. SPLENDA® No Calorie Sweetener. Johnson & Johnson. 20 Apr 2004. http://www.jnj.com/innovations/newfeatures/splenda.htm.

Walker, Barbara. The Little House Cookbook: Frontier Foods from Laura Ingalls Wilder's Classic Stories Harper Trophy, 1989.

Walker, Norman W. Fresh Vegetable and Fruit Juices. 1970. Prescott: Norwalk Press, 1978.

Wilson, James. Adrenal Fatigue. 2001. Petaluma: Smart Publications, 2001.

Notes

Notes

451070